Face Painting

and Dressing Up for Kids

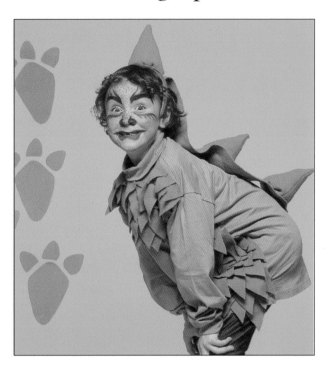

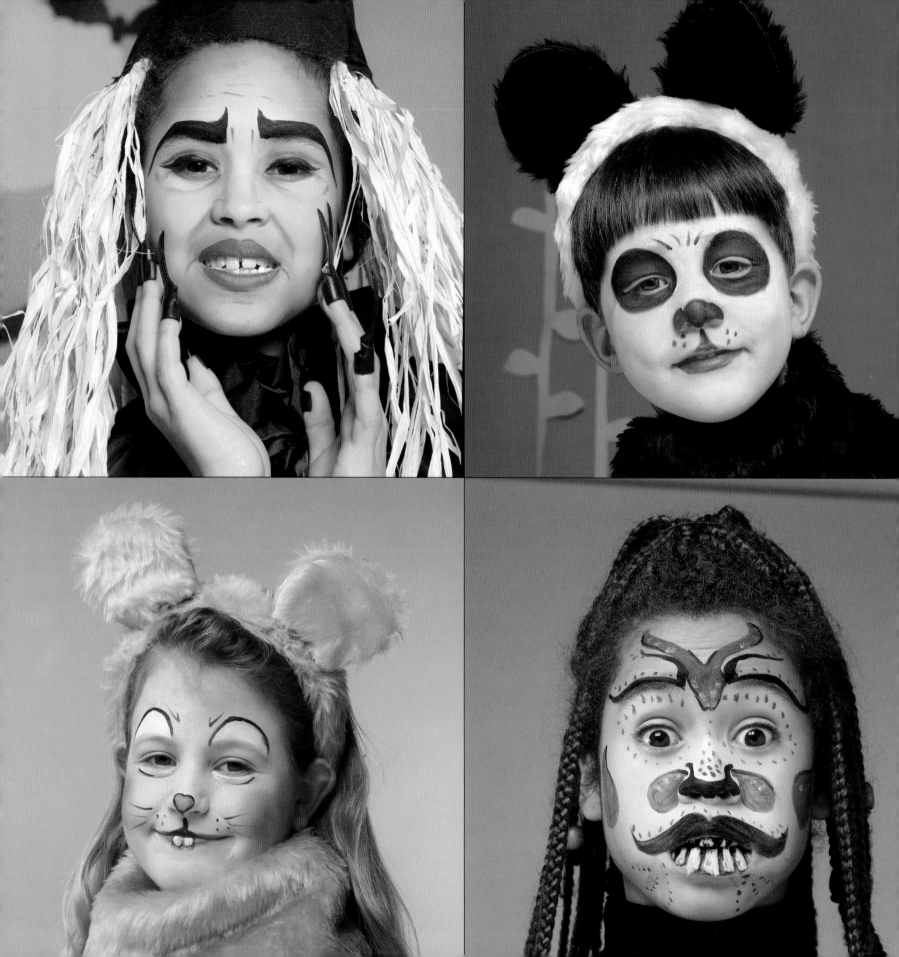

STEP-BY-STEP

Face Painting
and Dressing Up for Kids

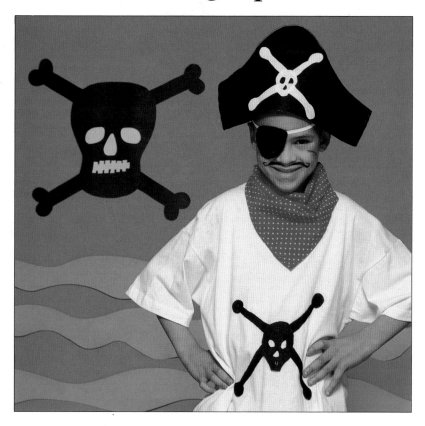

Petra Boase
face painting by Bettina Graham

photography by John Freeman

SMITHMARK

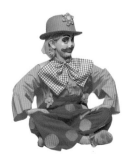

CONTENTS

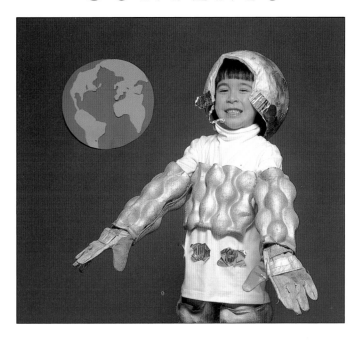

INTRODUCTION

Whether you are having a party, putting on a play or just having fun at home, dressing up and face painting provide great excitement and lots of laughs.

There are all sorts of different costume and face painting ideas for you to choose from in the book, but remember to read the instructions first and allow yourself enough time to make the costume. You don't want to be turning up to a party or performing in a play wearing a costume that is only half made!

In order to keep the costumes as inexpensive as possible, spend time looking in second-hand shops and flea markets for old clothes and fabric. These can then be cut up or altered according to the costume. Fabric paints are very useful if you wish to design your own patterns and motifs but remember to read the instructions properly before using them.

Before you start the face painting, make sure that your model is sitting comfortably and has a towel wrapped around his or her shoulders to protect his or her clothes. Keep any loose hair off the face with a hairband or a few hair clips. It is also a good idea to lay out all your paints and equipment on a table that is close by and have a mirror at hand so that your model can see how the design is evolving.

When you have finished making a costume or face painting, remember to clean up all your equipment and tidy it away neatly.

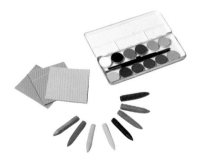

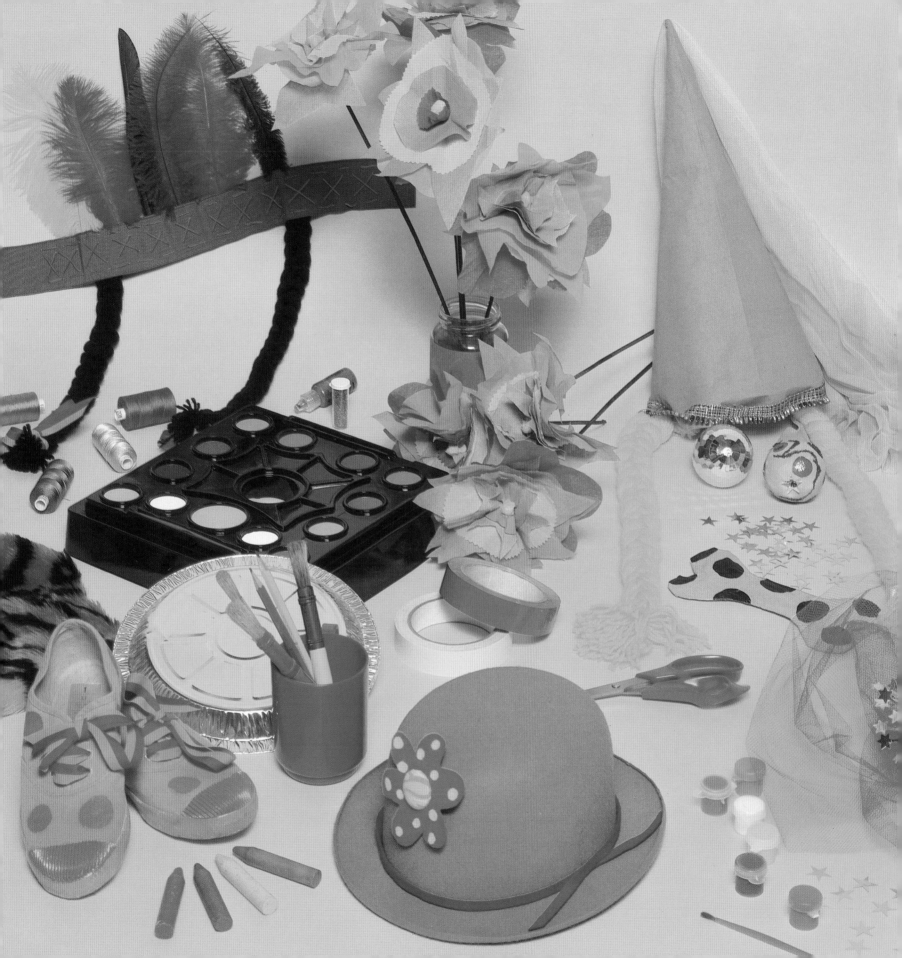

Materials and Equipment

These are a selection of the materials used in this book. If you can't find exactly the same materials, see if there is anything else you could substitute.

Baubles (balls)
These can be used to decorate headdresses and other accessories. Only use baubles made from plastic or paper.

Braid
This comes in a range of styles and widths and can be used to decorate clothes and accessories.

Buttons
Interesting buttons can be used as decoration.

Coloured adhesive tape
This strong tape can be used for fastening heavy materials. It also can be used for decoration.

Coloured paper
Heavy paper can be used for making hats and headdresses.

Covered elastic cord
This can be purchased from department stores and comes in different colours and strengths. It can be attached to hats to make them easier to wear.

Crepe and tissue paper
These can be used for decoration. They are quite fragile and are best suited to costumes that will only need to be worn once or twice.

Feathers
These can be bought from sewing shops and can be used to decorate hats and accessories.

Felt
This comes in a range of colours. It is easy to cut and won't fray.

Garden canes
These have many uses. Decorate one and turn it into a fairy's wand, or use several as the stems on a fun bunch of paper flowers.

Glitter
This can be glued on as decoration. If there is any left be sure to pour it back into the tube to use again.

Hairbands
These can be decorated to make a headdress or covered in fur to make a pair of ears.

Hessian (burlap)
This heavy cloth is perfect for costumes. When cut, the cloth may be frayed to make a fringe.

Metal kitchen scourers
These are made of soft metal and are used in the kitchen to clean pots and pans but they also make fun decorations.

Milliner's wire
This is covered with thread and is therefore safer to use than ordinary wire. You should still take care with the sharp ends, and cover them with tape.

Netting
This fabric is perfect for making light, airy skirts and wings. It is available in a wide range of colours from fabric shops.

Newspaper
Save old newspaper and use to protect surfaces when you are working or to make papier mâché.

Paintbrushes
Use a range of different sizes to apply paint and glue.

Paints
Use non-toxic paints to add details. If you don't have exactly the colour you want, try mixing paints together to make new ones.

Poppers (snaps)
These are quicker to add to a costume than buttons and buttonholes.

Ribbons
These come in a range of colours and patterns and can be used for making bows as decoration.

Safety pins
These can be taped onto the back of badges or used to help thread elastic through a waistband.

Sewing thread
Some of the costumes require basic sewing techniques. It is a good idea to match your sewing thread to your main material.

String
String can be used as a single fastener on an outfit, or can be used for hanging pendants.

Supermarket packaging
Boxes, egg cartons, and plastic and foil containers can all be used to make and decorate costumes.

Tin foil
This can be cut up or crumpled to create different decorative effects.

Tinsel
Save spare tinsel from the Christmas tree and use it to create sparkly accessories and details.

Wool
This can be used for making wigs and plaits (braids).

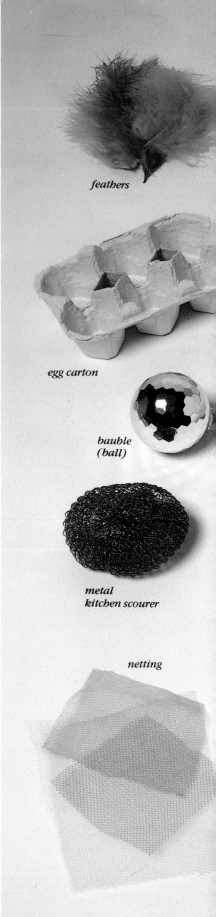

feathers

egg carton

bauble (ball)

metal kitchen scourer

netting

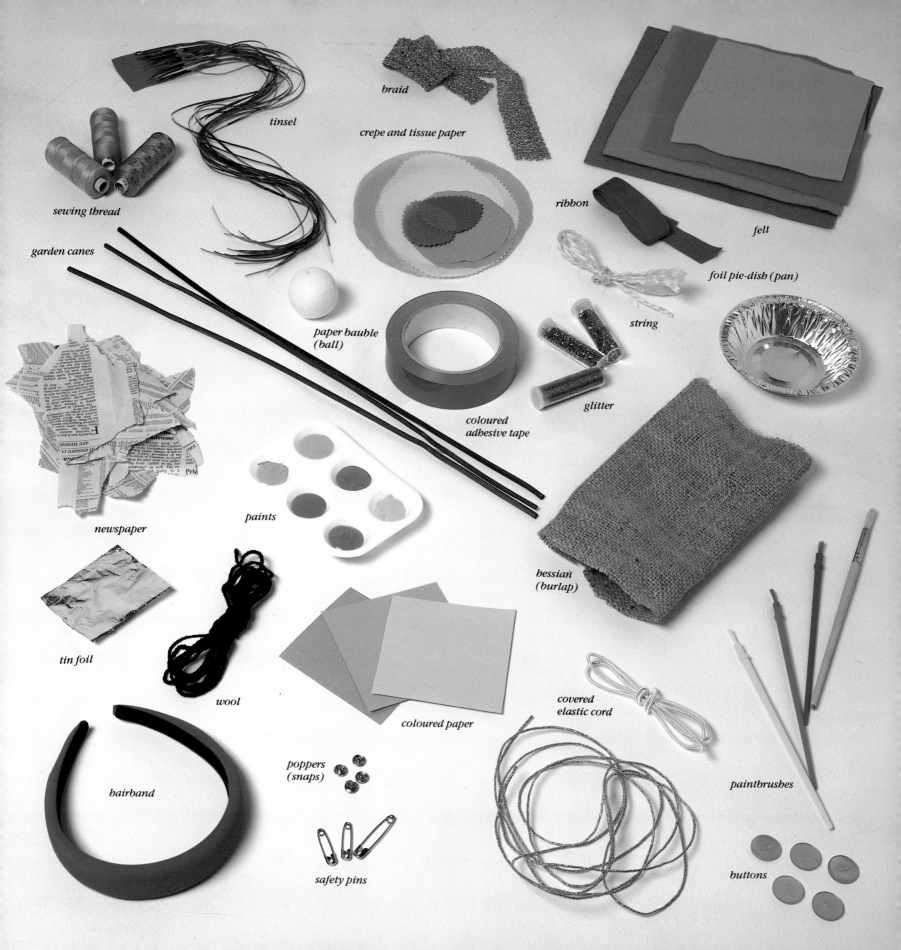

tinsel

braid

crepe and tissue paper

ribbon

felt

sewing thread

garden canes

paper bauble
(ball)

foil pie-dish (pan)

string

coloured
adhesive tape

glitter

newspaper

paints

hessian
(burlap)

tin foil

wool

coloured paper

covered
elastic cord

paintbrushes

hairband

poppers
(snaps)

safety pins

buttons

Face Painting Materials

There is an enormous range of face painting materials available at a range of different prices. Toy and novelty shops often stock a range of face paints, as well as theatrical suppliers.

Child's make-up kit
This is a good starter kit. It includes a bright range of coloured face paints, sponges, brushes, and a well for water. It is available from most toy shops.

Cleansing towels
These are ideal for removing the last traces of face paint.

Cold cream cleanser
Even though most water-based face paints come off with soap and water, you can also use a cream cleanser with soft tissues or cotton wool.

Cotton buds
These are used to apply and remove make-up around the eye.

Eyebrow brush
This is used for combing eyebrows and eyelashes.

Fake blood
This is great for special effects and can be purchased from theatrical and novelty shops.

Glitter gel
This comes in a range of colours and gives a sparkly finish. It can be purchased from costume shops.

Make-up brushes
These come in a range of sizes and shapes. It is a good idea to have different types to use for different effects. Wide brushes either have a flat or rounded edge and are used for large areas of modelling or for applying blusher, highlights or all-over powder. Medium brushes with a rounded edge are useful for modelling colour, while narrow brushes, either flat or pointed, are used for outlining and painting fine details and lips.

Make-up fixative
This is available from professional theatrical shops. It fixes the make-up, therefore making it last longer. Make sure the models eyes are closed when spraying it.

Make-up palette
This provides a range of solid, vibrant colours that give very good effects. You can mix colours together if the set you have doesn't provide the range of colours you require.

Make-up (eye-liner) pencils
These are used for drawing fine details on the face. They can also be used for outlining your basic design, if necessary.

Make-up pots
These are purchased from specialist theatrical shops. They are more expensive but are excellent quality and come in a wonderful range of colours.

Plastic palette
Use as a surface for mixing face paints together to achieve more subtle colours.

Soft tissue
Use with a dab of cold cream cleanser to remove make-up or for wiping off excess make-up from your brush.

Sponges
Covered sponges such as powder puffs are used for applying dry powders. Cellulose or latex sponges can be used slightly damp to give an even colour. Stipple sponges are made from soft plastic and are used for creating textured effects such as beard growth, animal skins and other effects.

Temple white
This is available from theatrical shops and is applied to the hair to give an aged effect.

Wax make-up crayons
If you do not mind a less professional finish, these are a good, inexpensive option. They give a less solid colour and the result is less long-lasting but they are often formulated for young children to use themselves.

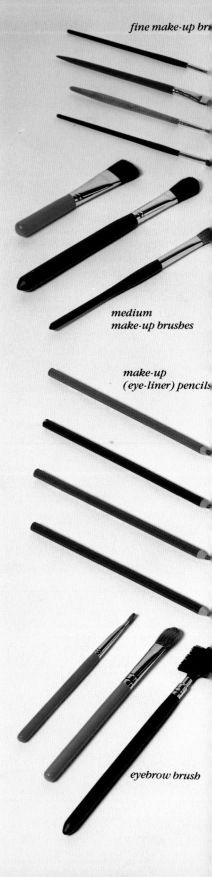

fine make-up br[ushes]

medium make-up brushes

make-up (eye-liner) pencils

eyebrow brush

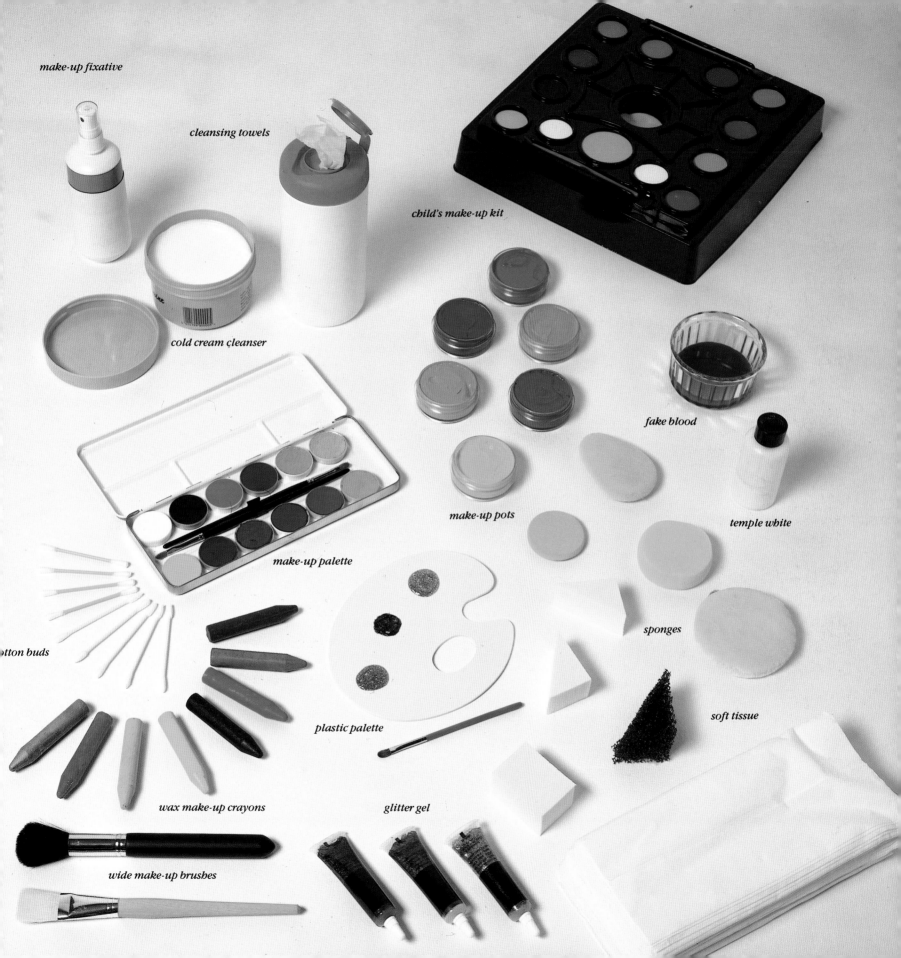

make-up fixative

cleansing towels

child's make-up kit

cold cream cleanser

fake blood

make-up palette

make-up pots

temple white

otton buds

sponges

plastic palette

soft tissue

wax make-up crayons

glitter gel

wide make-up brushes

TECHNIQUES

Making a Waistband

Elasticated waistbands make all costumes easy to put on and take off.

YOU WILL NEED
needle and thread or sewing machine
safety pin
elastic

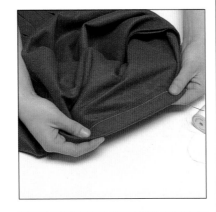

1 Fold over the waist and sew a line of stitches to make a tube. Leave a gap to thread the elastic through.

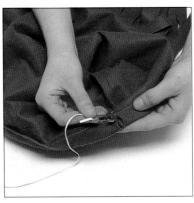

2 Attach a safety pin to the end of the elastic and thread it through the tube until it comes out the other end.

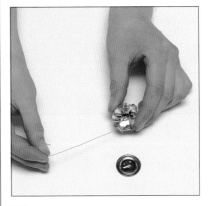

3 Pull the two ends of elastic to gather the waist to the right size and tie a knot. Sew up the opening in the tube.

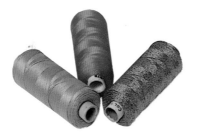

Covering a Button

By covering buttons you can choose your own fabric to match the outfit. The clown costume includes lots of colourful buttons.

YOU WILL NEED
fabric
scissors
self-covering button
needle and thread

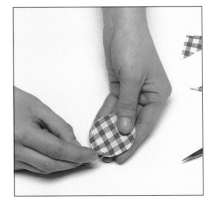

1 Cut out a circle of fabric twice as wide as the button. Sew a line of running stitches around the edge of circle.

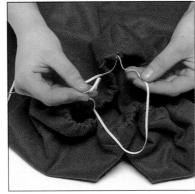

2 Open the button and place the front on the circle of fabric. Pull the threads to gather them up around the button.

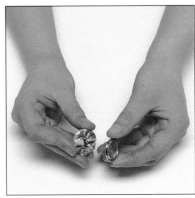

3 Place the back on the button.

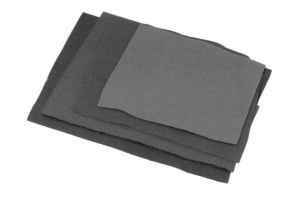

Decorative Stitches

These stitches can add a finishing touch to an outfit, whether adding colourful details in thread, or sewing on fabric shapes.

YOU WILL NEED
needle and thread

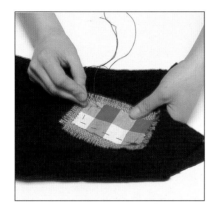

1 Running stitch is useful for sewing on patches and other shapes. You can make the stitches as long or as short as you like.

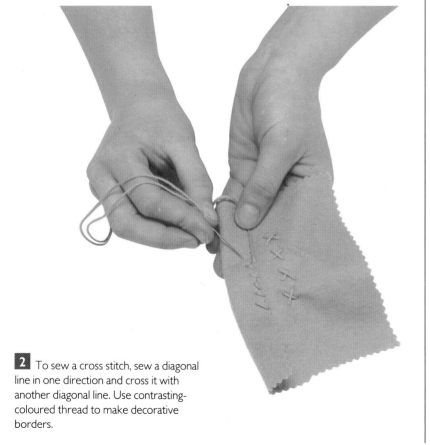

2 To sew a cross stitch, sew a diagonal line in one direction and cross it with another diagonal line. Use contrasting-coloured thread to make decorative borders.

Making your own Pantaloons

Decorate the pantaloons according to the character required. These basic pantaloons can be used for the pirate and genie costumes.

YOU WILL NEED
2 metres/2 yards fabric
pattern, enlarged from the template section
scissors
needle and thread or sewing machine
safety pin
elastic

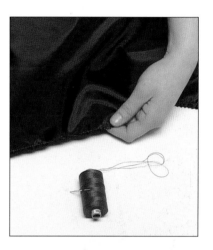

1 Fold the fabric in half, with the right sides facing, and place the pattern on the fold of the fabric. Cut out two identical pieces. Keep each piece of the pantaloon folded in half with the right sides facing and sew along the inside leg with a 5 mm/¼ in seam allowance.

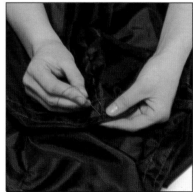

2 Turn one leg piece right side out and place it inside the other leg, matching up the raw edges. Stitch the two pieces together. Turn the legs right side out. Fold over the waist of the pantaloons and sew a double line of stitching to make a tube for the elastic to go through. Leave a gap to thread the elastic through. Do the same around the bottom of each pantaloon leg.

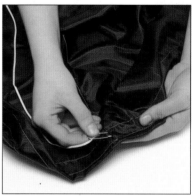

3 Attach the safety pin to one end of the elastic and tie a knot at the end. Thread the elastic through the tube. Do the same with each pantaloon leg. Sew up the gaps in the tubes.

Papier Mâché

Papier mâché can be used for all kinds of things. In this book it has been used to make jewellery, accessories and helmets.

YOU WILL NEED
PVA (white) glue
bowl
water
paintbrush
newspaper
cardboard cut in the shape you want
    to make, or balloon
petroleum jelly (optional)

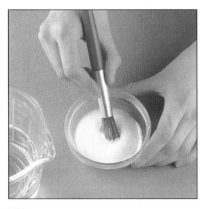

1 For the paste, pour some PVA (white) glue into a bowl and add water. Mix the two together with a paintbrush. The mixture should not be too runny.

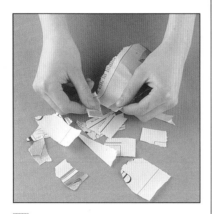

2 Tear up sheets of newspaper into small pieces. Dip the pieces one at a time into the glue and stick them onto the cardboard shape.

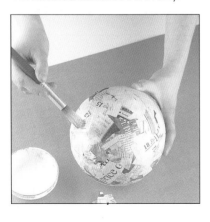

3 Cover the cardboard shape with approximately three layers of paper and leave it to dry thoroughly. If you are covering a balloon, apply water or petroleum jelly to the surface and then the layers of paper. This will stop the shape sticking to the balloon when you pop it.

Tracing a Template

Some of the projects in this book use templates. To transfer the template to a piece of card simply follow these instructions.

YOU WILL NEED
tracing paper
soft pencil
cardboard or paper
scissors

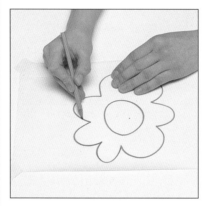

1 Place a piece of tracing paper over the template and draw around the shape using a pencil. The outline should be dark and heavy.

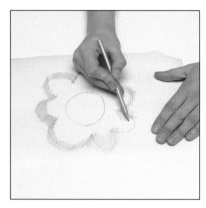

2 Take the tracing paper off the template and turn it over. Rub over the traced image with the pencil on the reverse side of the tracing paper.

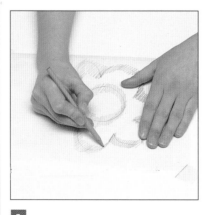

3 Place the tracing paper on a piece of cardboard or paper with the rubbed pencil side facing down. Draw over the lines you have made with the pencil to transfer the picture.

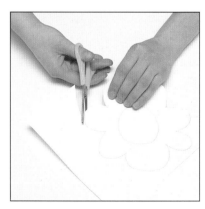

4 Cut out the template, and use as a pattern for costumes or accessories.

Applying Eye Make-up and Handling the Brush

Successful face painting is all about feeling confident handling the brush. Practise brush strokes until you feel confident enough to attempt a complete design. If you are not happy with what you have done, simply remove the make-up with soap and water or a cream cleanser, and start again.

YOU WILL NEED
water-based face paints
fine make-up brush
tissue

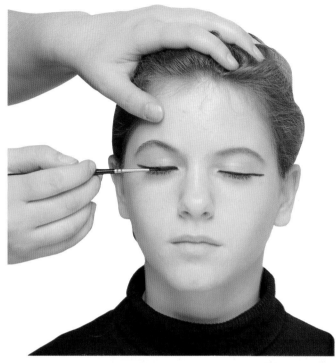

1 Ask the model to close her eyes and paint a straight line across each eyelid. Ensure the brush is not too wet, and do not work too close to the eyelashes. If the make-up should get into the eyes, wash with warm water immediately. You may want to rest on the model to give you a steadier hand.

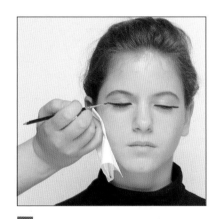

2 You can also support your hand on the model's cheek, resting on a piece of tissue to help you paint a smooth straight line. After some practice you will find out what is most comfortable.

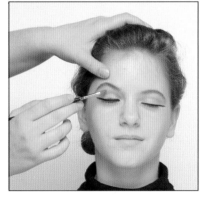

3 When shading above the model's eye, the model should look down at the floor. You may need to wait a few minutes for the make-up to dry before moving onto the next stage.

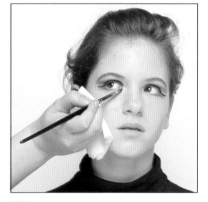

4 When shading under the model's eye, support your hand on her cheek, resting on a piece of tissue. Ask the model to look up while you apply the make-up, and start at the inner corner of the eye.

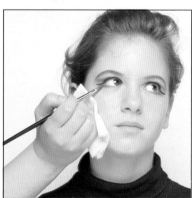

5 Continue to the outer corner, making an even, sweeping motion beyond the outer corner of the eye. This will enhance the eyes, and give a dramatic finish.

Applying a Base

An evenly applied, well-modelled base is the foundation for successful face-painting effects. Experiment with different colours, blended directly onto the face, to change the model's appearance.

YOU WILL NEED
make-up sponge
water-based face paints

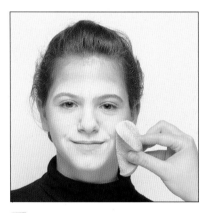

1 Using a damp sponge, begin to apply the base colour over the face. To avoid streaks or patchiness, make sure the sponge is not too wet.

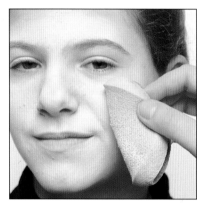

2 Make sure the base is applied evenly over the face and fill in any patchy areas.

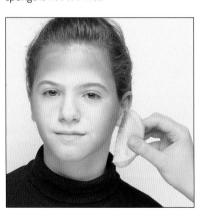

3 Using a contrasting colour, sponge around the edge of the face.

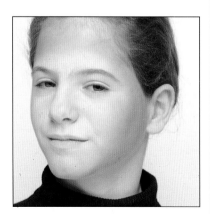

4 Blend the colours together for an even finish. Always make sure the base colours are dry before you start to decorate the face with other colours.

Shading

Shading can change the shape of your model's face dramatically.

YOU WILL NEED
powder face paints
soft make-up brush

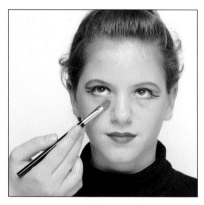

1 When shading under the model's eyes, ask her to look up so that the area becomes smooth and easy to work on. This also stops the model from blinking as you work.

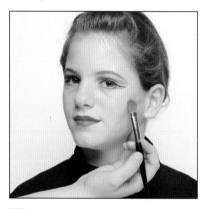

2 To exaggerate the shape of the model's face, shade each cheekbone with blusher or dark powder face paint.

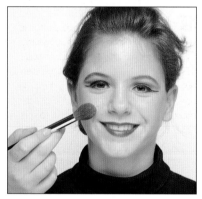

3 To shade the whole face, use a large soft brush.

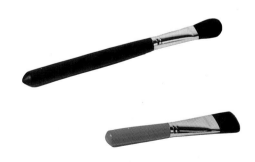

Painting Lips

YOU WILL NEED
fine lipstick brush
water-based face paints

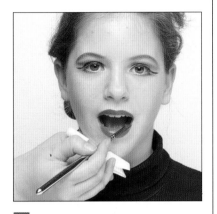

1 Using a fine lipstick brush, paint the lips. Ask the model to close her mouth as this makes the muscles firmer and easier to outline. Then ask the model to open her mouth to fill in the corners. You may need to wait a few seconds to allow the make-up to dry before going on to the next stage.

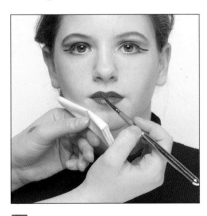

2 Rest your hand on the model's chin, on a piece of tissue or a powder puff. This will help you to paint an even outline around the lips. You might want to experiment with using a different colour for the outline, or extending the line beyond the natural curve of the model's mouth to create a different shape.

Ageing the Face

You can make even the young look very old with this technique.

YOU WILL NEED
water-based face paints
fine make-up brush
wide make-up brush

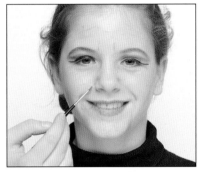

1 To find where wrinkles occur naturally, ask the model to frown. This will show where lines will occur with age. Apply fine lines of make-up in these areas. Ask the model to smile, and apply a fine line starting at either side of the nose, down the fold of the cheek.

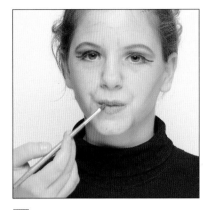

2 Ask your model to purse her lips, and apply fine lines around the mouth, within the natural folds.

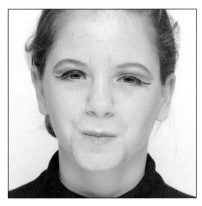

3 Finish by giving a light dusting of a lighter coloured base with a wide brush on the cheeks and temples.

Removing Make-up

Most face paints will come off with soap and water. If soap is too drying, or if some colours persist, you may want to remove make-up as follows.

YOU WILL NEED
cold cream cleanser
cotton wool ball or soft tissues

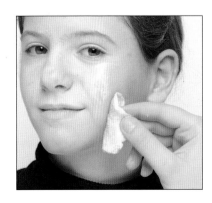

1 Pour the cream onto a damp cotton wool ball or tissue and gently rub the make-up off the face. Use a clean tissue or your fingers to apply more cold cream cleanser.

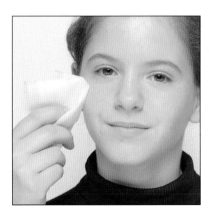

2 If desired, give a final cleanse with soap and water, and dry by patting the face with a soft towel.

Making a Tail

This tail was made to go with the spotted dog outfit. You can make a tail for a cat or tiger in the same way.

YOU WILL NEED
old pair of children's black tights
scissors
newspaper
elastic
needle and thread
felt
fabric glue

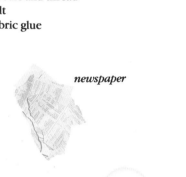

newspaper

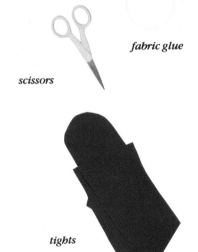

fabric glue

scissors

tights

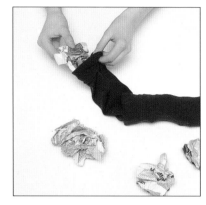

1 Cut one leg off the pair of tights. Scrunch up balls of newspaper and fill up the leg until it is quite firm.

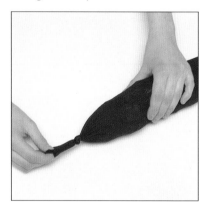

2 Tie a knot at the end of the leg.

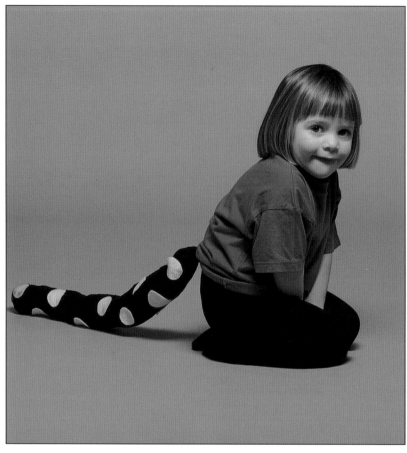

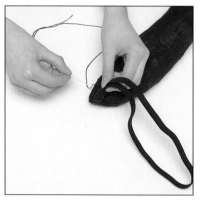

3 Measure your waist so you know how much elastic you need. Sew the elastic in a loop onto the knotted end of the tail.

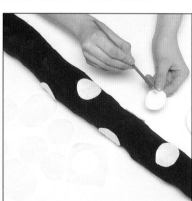

4 This tail is for the spotted dog so it has been decorated with spots of felt glued on with fabric glue. You could always paint on a different design using fabric paints.

Making Ears

These ears add a cuddly touch to any of the animal outfits. You can adjust the size of the ears and choose material to suit the animal.

YOU WILL NEED
hairband
tape measure
fake fur
scissors
needle and thread
felt
fabric glue (optional)
template for ears
cardboard
pencil

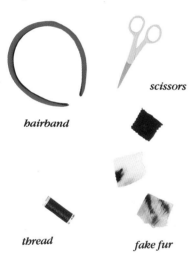

scissors

hairband

thread

fake fur

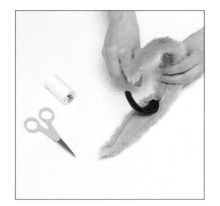

1 Measure the length of the hairband with a tape measure. Cut out a piece of fur to fit, allowing an extra 2 cm/1 in at each end for folding over. Sew the fur onto the hairband as shown.

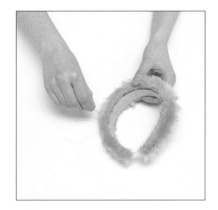

2 Cut out a piece of felt to fit the inside of the hairband and sew or glue it on.

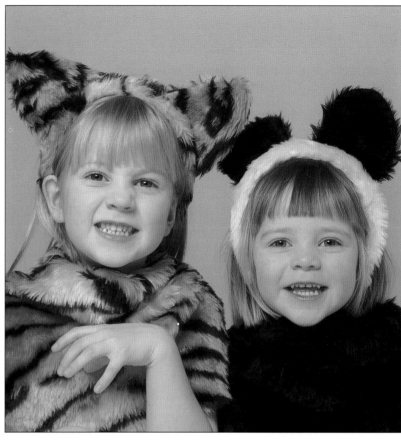

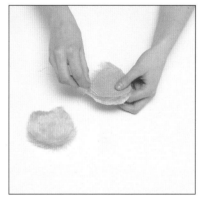

3 Trace the appropriate template from the back of the book onto a piece of cardboard and draw around the cardboard on the reverse side of the fur. You will need two pieces of fur for each ear. Place the two pieces of fur together with the right sides facing and sew round, leaving a gap to turn the right sides out.

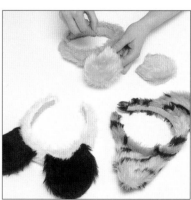

4 Sew the ears onto the hairband, making sure they are in the correct position.

Cat

Use the instructions given previously in this chapter to make a pair of black furry ears. Dress up in a black catsuit and you will be the most glamorous, sleek pussy cat in town.

YOU WILL NEED
make-up sponge
water-based face paints
medium make-up brush
fine make-up brush
thick make-up brush
blusher

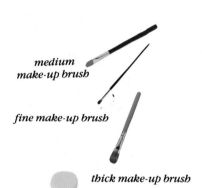

medium make-up brush

fine make-up brush

thick make-up brush

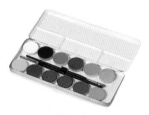

make-up sponge

water-based face paints

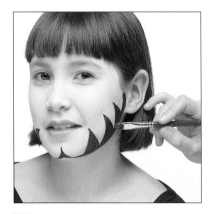

1 Using a damp sponge, apply a white base over the whole face. Using a medium brush, paint a border of black spikes around the edge of the face. You might find it easier to paint the outline first and then fill it in.

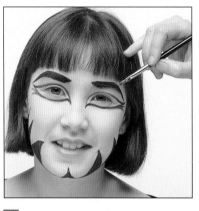

2 Paint a black outline around the eyes as shown and paint over the eyebrows.

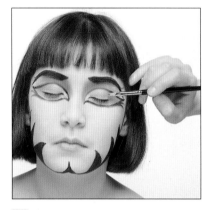

3 Making sure the model's eyes are closed, fill in the eyelids and inside the black outline with a bright colour. This is a very delicate part of the face, so take care, and do not apply make-up too close to the eyelashes. Paint above the eyes.

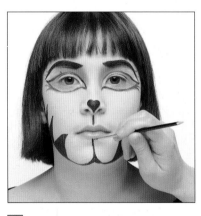

4 Using a fine brush, paint a heart shape on the tip of the nose and a thin line joining the nose to the chin, avoiding the mouth.

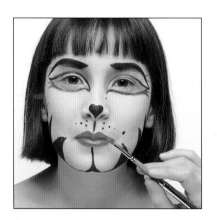

5 Paint the lips a bright colour and paint black whisker spots under the nose.

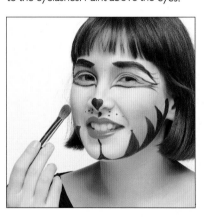

6 Using a thick brush, dust each cheek with blusher.

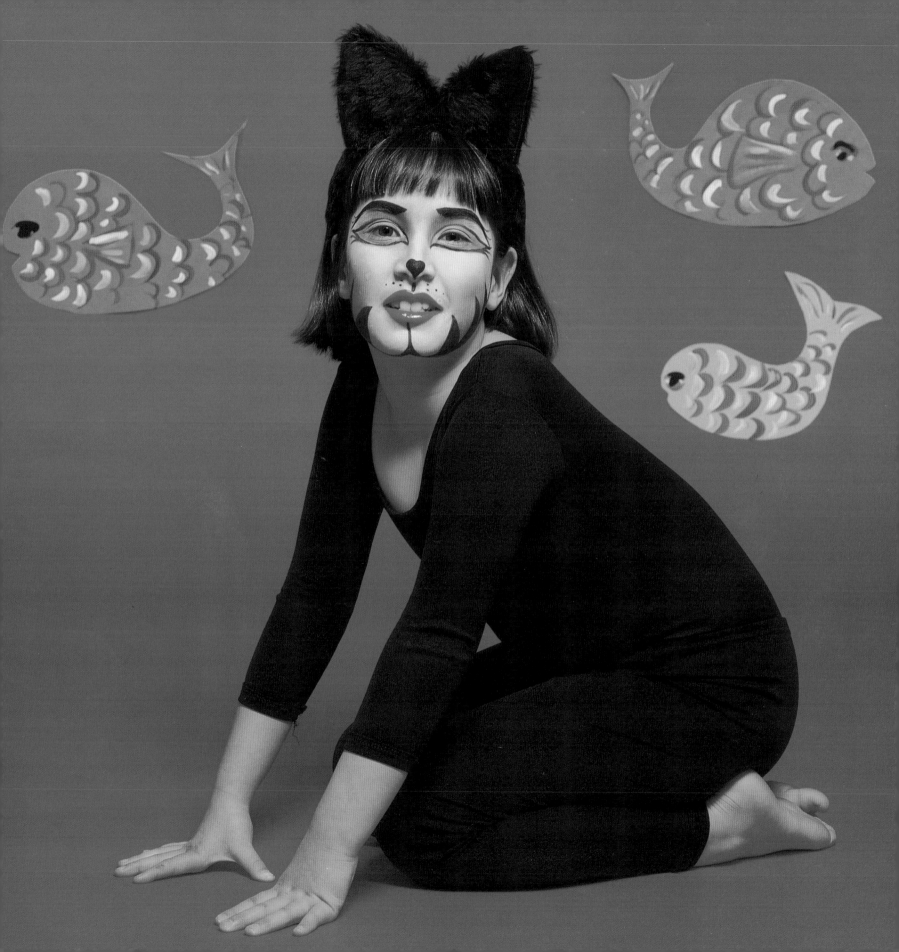

Animal Collar

This elegant and stylish collar will make any animal look a million dollars.

YOU WILL NEED
tape measure
black velvet ribbon
scissors
silver fabric or cardboard
fabric glue
sequins
needle and thread
popper (snap) or hook and eye

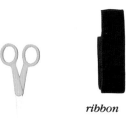

scissors

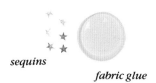

ribbon

sequins

fabric glue

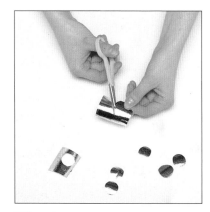

1 Ask an adult or a friend to help measure your neck with a tape measure so that you know how long you need the ribbon to be, and cut it to this length. For the decoration, cut out six dots from silver fabric or cardboard.

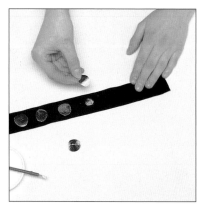

2 Glue the spots onto the ribbon at equal distances from each other, making sure there is enough room between each one for a sequin. Leave them to dry.

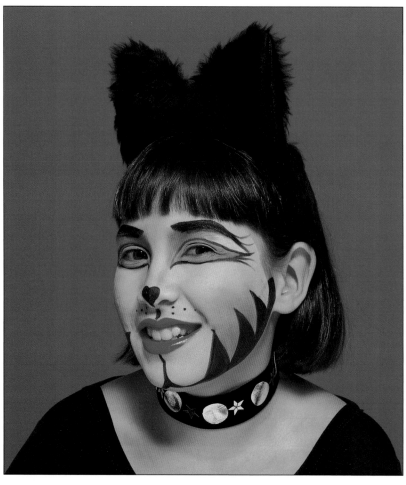

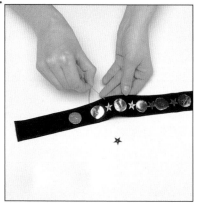

3 Sew on a sequin in between each silver spot.

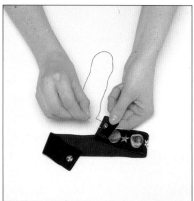

4 Fold the ends of the ribbon over and secure them down with a dab of glue. Sew on the fasteners and the collar is ready to wear.

Papier Mâché Pendant and Badge

These fun pieces of jewellery will add the finishing touch to your outfit.

YOU WILL NEED
templates for dog bone badge and fish
    pendant
cardboard
scissors
PVA (white) glue
bowl
water
newspaper
paints
paintbrush
brooch pins
tin foil
hole puncher
ribbon

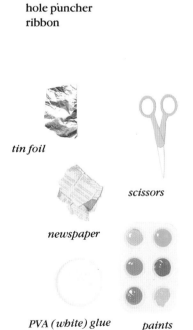

tin foil

scissors

newspaper

PVA (white) glue   *paints*

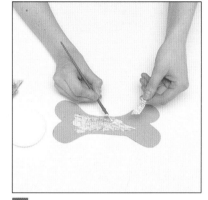

1 Using the template for the dog bone badge, cut out a bone shape from a piece of cardboard. Cover the cardboard with layers of papier mâché as described in the introduction. To make the badge slightly three-dimensional, roll up small balls of newspaper and stick them onto the bone. Cover them with strips of newspaper for a smooth finish. Leave the bone to dry.

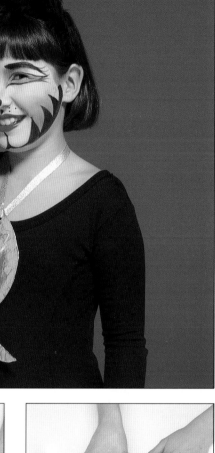

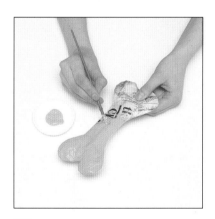

2 Paint the bone a bright colour and, when the paint has dried, add large dots in a contrasting colour. Leave to dry.

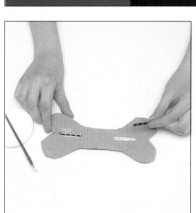

3 Using PVA (white) glue, stick two brooch pins onto the back of the badge. Leave the glue to harden before trying on the badge.

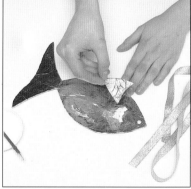

4 Make the fish pendant in the same way as the bone except, instead of painting it, cover the fish and the fin in foil. You will need a hole puncher to make the hole for the ribbon.

Tiger

For a complete look, dress up in an outfit made from fake tiger fur and use the instructions at the beginning of this chapter to make a pair of matching furry ears.

YOU WILL NEED
make-up sponge
water-based face paints
medium make-up brush
fine make-up brush

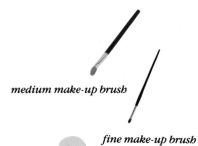

medium make-up brush

fine make-up brush

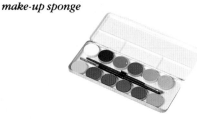

make-up sponge

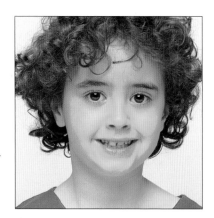

water-based face paints

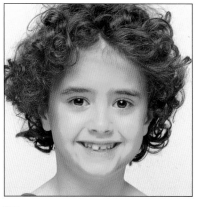

1 Using a damp sponge, apply the base colour over the face.

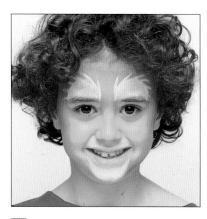

2 Rinse the sponge, then stipple a darker shade of paint around the edge of the face as shown.

3 Sponge the chin and the area above the mouth white. Using a medium brush, paint the area around the eyes white as shown. You might find it easier to paint the outline first and then fill it in.

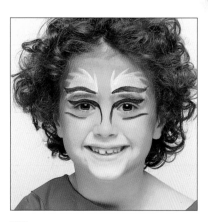

4 Using a medium brush, paint on the black markings around each eye, as shown, making sure each side is the same.

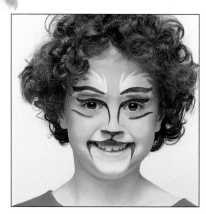

5 Using a fine brush, paint the tip of the nose black and paint a thin black line from the centre of the nose to the top lip. Paint the top lip black and extend the line at each corner of the mouth, stopping half-way down the chin.

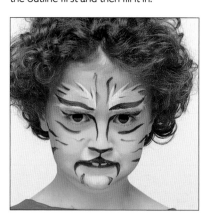

6 For the rest of the markings, paint brushstrokes of colour across the face. To keep the design symmetrical, finish one side of the face first and then copy the design onto the other side.

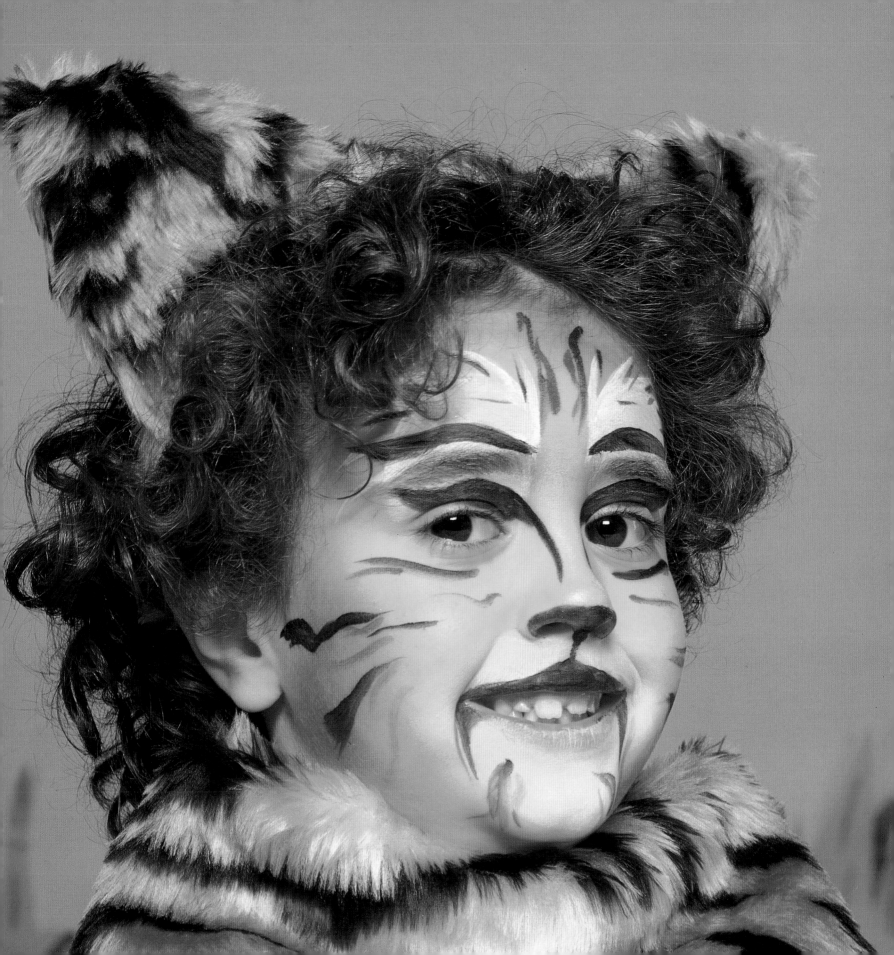

Lion

The wilder your hair is the fiercer you will look. Try roaring and snarling in a mirror to see what different expressions you can make, but try not to frighten any of your friends or family. Complete the look by making a pair of ears as for the cat costume.

YOU WILL NEED
make-up sponge
water-based face paints
natural sea sponge
medium make-up brush
fine make-up brush or make-up (eye-
    liner) pencil
lipstick brush
thick make-up brush

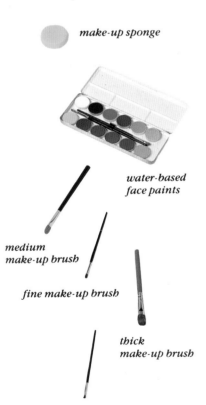

make-up sponge

*water-based
face paints*

*medium
make-up brush*

fine make-up brush

*thick
make-up brush*

lipstick brush

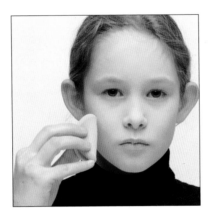

1 Using a damp sponge, apply the base colour over the face.

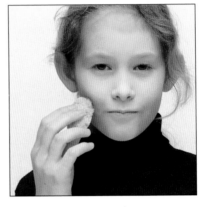

2 Using a natural sponge, dab a darker shade around the edge of the face as shown.

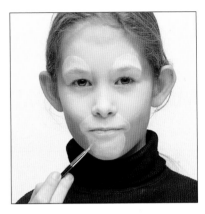

3 Using a medium brush, apply white make-up over each eyebrow to form an almost circular shape. Colour the area around the mouth and chin white.

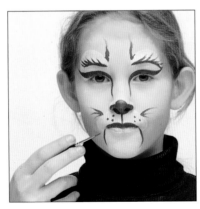

4 Study the picture carefully so that you know where to paint the markings on the face. You might find it easier to outline some of them with a fine brush or make-up (eye-liner) pencil first and then fill them in. Only paint the top lip at this stage.

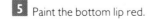

5 Paint the bottom lip red.

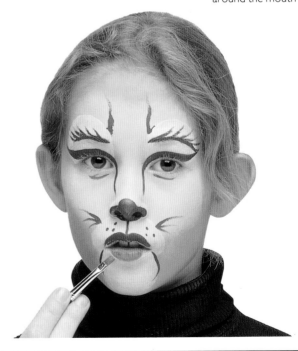

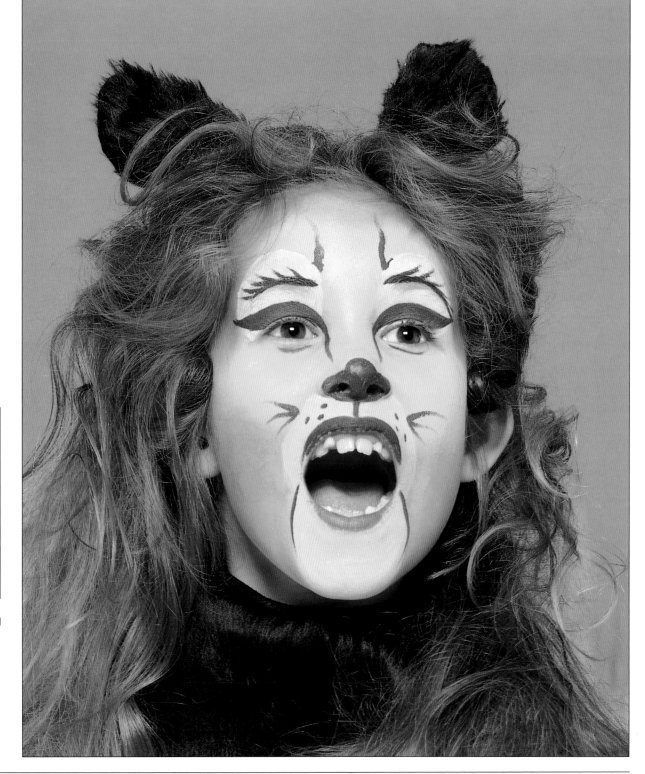

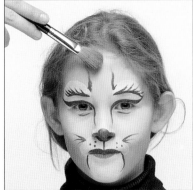

6 Using a thick brush, dust the nose and centre of the forehead with a shade of brown. Use the template for the cat ears to make some lion ears to finish off your costume.

Spotted Dog

This funny dog's outfit is easy to make. Simply cut out circles of felt and stick them onto a pair of leggings and a T-shirt using fabric glue. Use the template and the instructions provided earlier to make a pair of spotted ears and a tail to match.

YOU WILL NEED
make-up sponge
water-based face paints
fine make-up brush
medium make-up brush

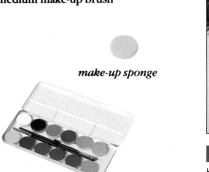

make-up sponge

water-based face paints

fine make-up brush

medium make-up brush

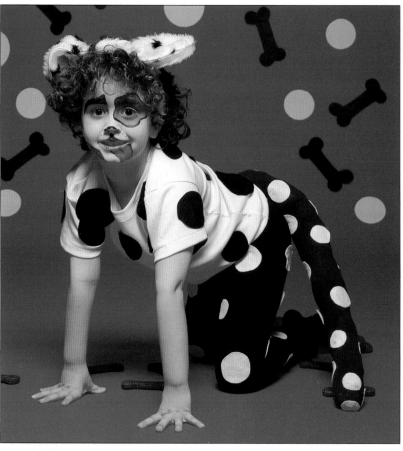

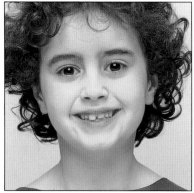

1 Using a damp sponge, apply a white base colour over the face. Gently sponge a slightly darker shade around the eyes.

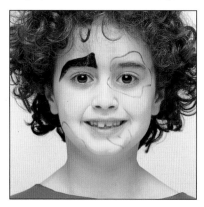

2 Paint one eyebrow black and, using a fine make-up brush, paint a wiggly outline around the other eye to make a patch. Paint another patch outline on the side of the face. Paint the outline for a droopy tongue below the bottom lip.

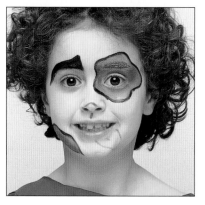

3 Using a medium brush fill in the patches grey and outline them in black. Draw the outline for the nose and a line joining the nose to the mouth.

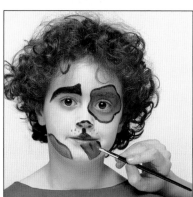

4 Fill in the tongue red and outline in black. Paint a short black line along the centre of the tongue. Fill in the tip of the nose pink and add a thick black line where the nose joins the mouth. Paint the centre of the top lip black. Paint black whisker spots under the nose.

Rabbit

This adorable little bunny is dressed all in white. As well as using the instructions provided earlier to make a pair of furry ears, you could also make a fluffy tail from cotton wool and stick it onto the T-shirt.

YOU WILL NEED
make-up sponge
water-based face paints
black make-up (eye-liner) pencil
medium make-up brush
pink blusher (optional)
fine make-up brush

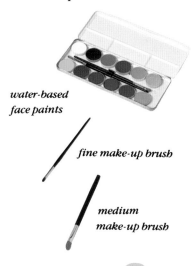

water-based face paints

fine make-up brush

medium make-up brush

make-up sponge

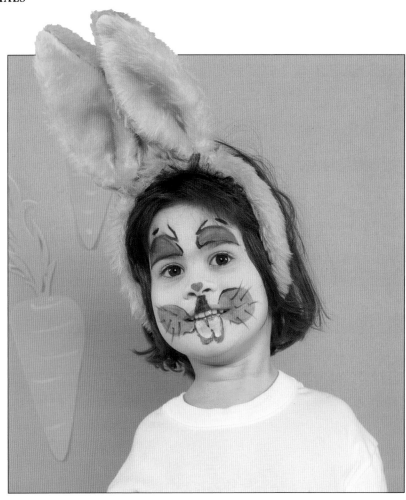

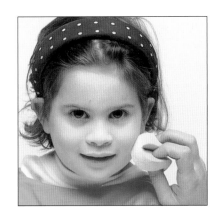

1 Using a damp sponge, apply a white base over the face.

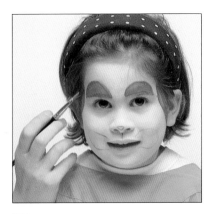

2 Using a black make-up (eye-liner) pencil draw a heart on the tip of the nose, a circular outline above each eyebrow, a line joining the nose to the mouth and a circle on each cheek. Using a medium brush, fill in the marked area above the eyebrows grey.

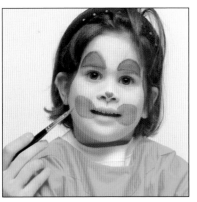

3 Paint the heart at the tip of the nose red and paint the cheeks pink with water-based face paints or pink blusher.

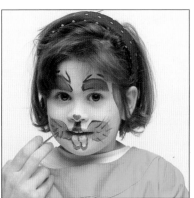

4 Using a fine brush, draw the outline of the teeth over the bottom lip and fill them in with white make-up. Using a medium brush, paint the line joining the nose to the mouth black. Paint black whiskers above each eyebrow and on each cheek.

Bumble Bee

Buzz around in this striped outfit. Why not paint a pair of tights or leggings in the same style?

YOU WILL NEED
yellow T-shirt
newspaper
black fabric paint
paintbrush
paints
hairband
paper baubles (balls)
scissors
milliner's wire
needle and thread
black felt
glue
black cardboard
pencil
needle and thread

FOR THE FACE
make-up sponge
water-based face paints
medium make-up brush

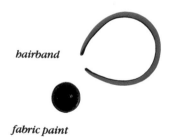
hairband

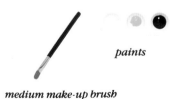
fabric paint

paints

medium make-up brush

glue

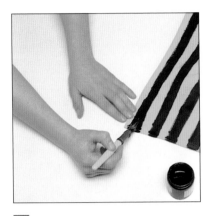

1 Place the T-shirt on a flat, well-covered surface. Fill the T-shirt with flat pieces of newspaper. Paint black lines across the T-shirt and on the arms and leave the paint to dry. Turn the T-shirt over to the other side and continue painting the lines.

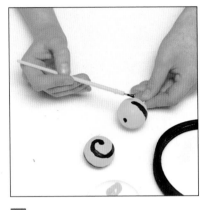

2 For the antennae, first paint the hairband black and leave the paint to dry. Paint the paper baubles (balls) yellow and, when the paint has dried, paint a black line around each one.

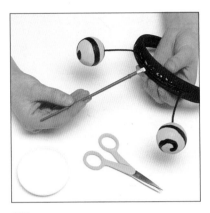

3 Cut a length of wire, approximately 45 cm/18 in long. Bend the wire to fit the hairband, making sure each piece of wire that will support the bauble is the same length. Sew the wire onto the hairband and glue a strip of black felt over the wire for extra support. Secure the baubles onto the ends of the wire.

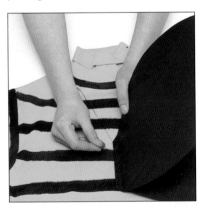

4 Fold a piece of black cardboard in half and draw the shape of a wing, so that, when it is cut out and the paper is opened out, you will have two identical wings that are joined together. Sew the wings along the fold onto the back of the T-shirt.

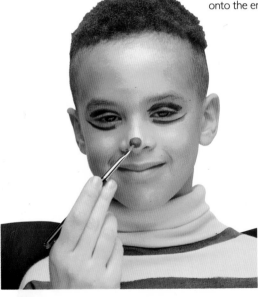

5 For the face, use a damp sponge to apply a yellow base. Using a medium brush, paint a black line on the eyelids and under each eye. Paint a black spot on the tip of the nose.

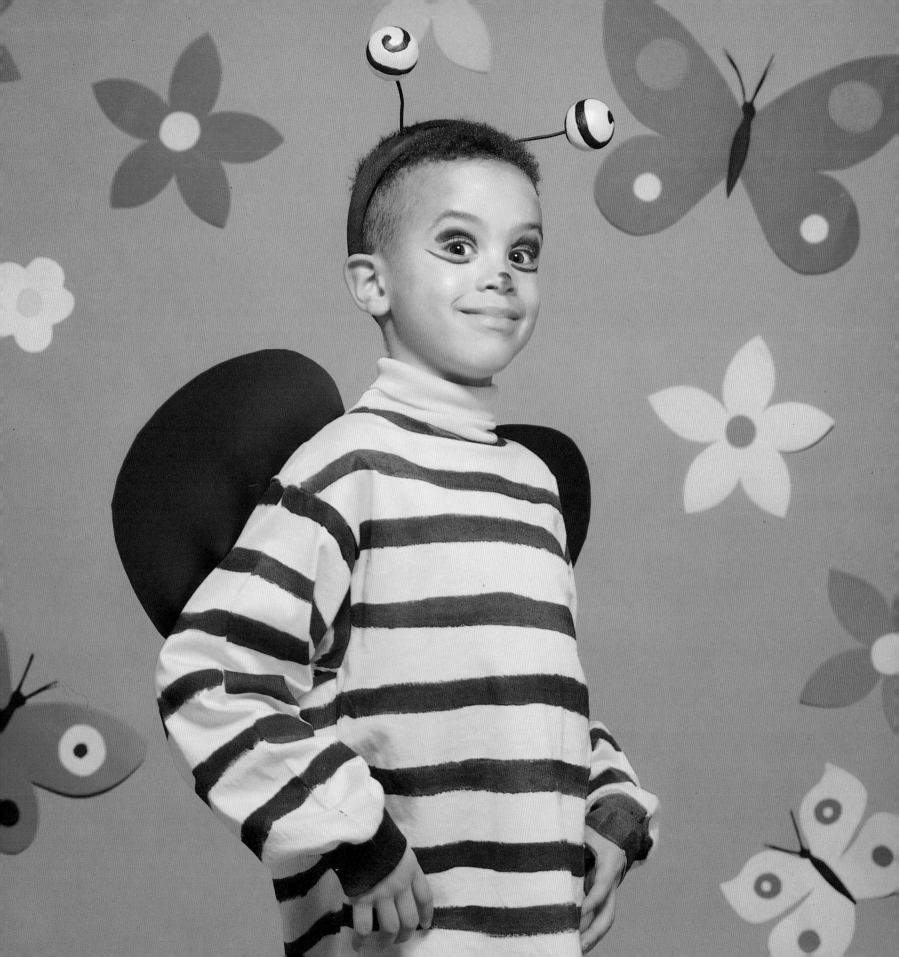

Butterfly

When you wear this pretty outfit, gently move your arms to make the wings flap.

YOU WILL NEED
2.5 metres/2½ yards milliner's wire
scissors
adhesive tape
coloured netting
needle and embroidery thread
smaller pieces of different coloured
    netting
silver or gold elastic cord
hairband
2 paper baubles (balls)
paints
paintbrush
glue
glitter
felt
leotard and tights

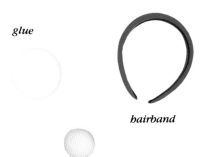

glue

hairband

paper bauble (ball)

glitter   *netting*

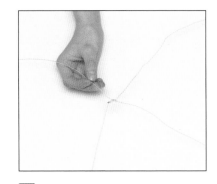

1 Cut a piece of milliner's wire approximately 2 metres/2 yards long. Bend the two ends together to make a big circle. For extra safety you can secure the ends with a piece of adhesive tape. Pinch the two sides of the wire circle together and twist. The wire should now resemble a figure-of-eight.

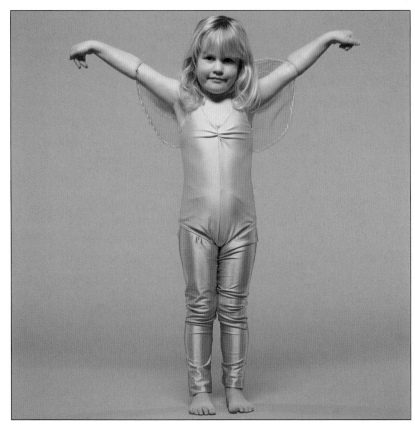

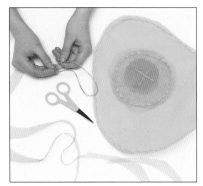

2 Place the wire frame between two pieces of coloured netting. Sew the netting onto the wire frame using a brightly coloured embroidery thread. Trim away any excess net. Cut out circles of different coloured netting and sew them onto each wing. To support the wings you will need to thread a loop of elastic cord onto the outside of each wing for the arms to slip through.

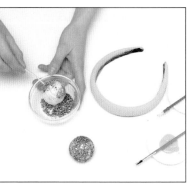

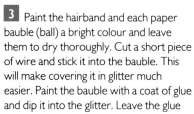

3 Paint the hairband and each paper bauble (ball) a bright colour and leave them to dry thoroughly. Cut a short piece of wire and stick it into the bauble. This will make covering it in glitter much easier. Paint the bauble with a coat of glue and dip it into the glitter. Leave the glue to dry.

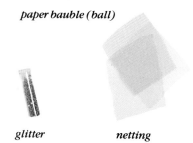

4 Cut another length of wire for the antennae, measuring 45 cm/18 in. Bend the wire to fit the hairband, making sure each end of wire is the same length. Fasten the wire to the hairband with glue and glue on a piece of felt for support. Decorate the hairband with glitter. Secure the baubles onto the ends of the wire. Complete the costume by wearing a leotard and pair of tights.

Mouse

Use the template and the instructions provided earlier to make a pair of furry mouse ears. Beware of cats and owls when you are wearing this costume as one of their favourite meals is little mice!

YOU WILL NEED
make-up sponge
water-based face paints
black make-up (eye-liner) pencil
medium make-up brush
thick make-up brush
pink blusher
fine make-up brush

make-up sponge

water-based face paints

fine make-up brush

medium make-up brush

thick make-up brush

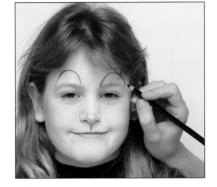

1 Using a damp sponge, apply a base coat of white over the face. With a black make-up (eye-liner) pencil, mark a pair of eyebrows above the model's own. Draw the outline of a heart on the tip of the nose and draw a line joining the nose to the mouth.

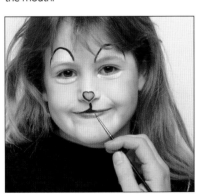

2 Using a medium brush, paint the area under the drawn eyebrows white. Apply more white underneath the model's eyes. Paint the heart pink and the outlines of the eyebrows and the heart black. Paint a line that joins the nose to the mouth and continue the line onto the centre of the top lip, forming a triangle.

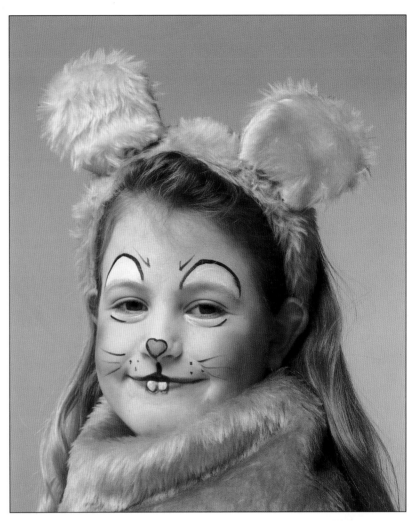

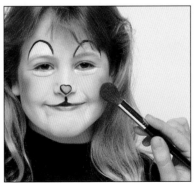

3 Using a thick brush, dust pink blusher onto each cheek.

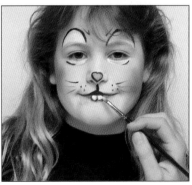

4 Using a fine brush, paint the black outline of the teeth over the bottom lip. Fill in the teeth white. Paint on a few black whisker spots and whiskers.

Owl

In this design, large yellow owl eyes are painted onto your eyelids, so when your eyes are closed, it looks as though they are wide open.

YOU WILL NEED
thick make-up brush
water-based face paints
medium make-up brush
fine make-up brush
hair spray
hair clips

medium make-up brush

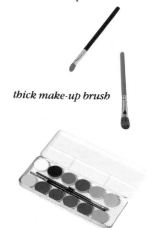

thick make-up brush

water-based face paints

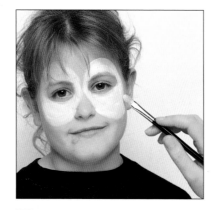

1 Using a thick brush, paint a white area around each eye, leaving bare the area immediately surrounding the eye.

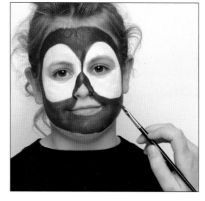

2 Paint the rest of the face brown, except for the mouth, the upper lip and the tip of the nose.

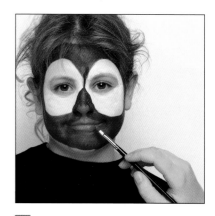

3 Using a medium brush, apply red to the tip of the nose, the upper lip and the mouth.

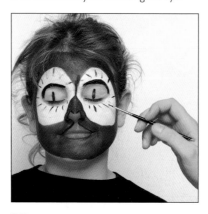

4 Making sure the brush is not too wet, gently paint yellow on the eyelids and around the eye. Do not apply too close to the eyelashes. Using a fine brush, paint a black stripe across the top of each eyelid and a short stripe down the centre. Paint a black line around the red nose and mouth area and black streaks around the eye area.

5 Add feathery streaks around the eye area in yellow and white.

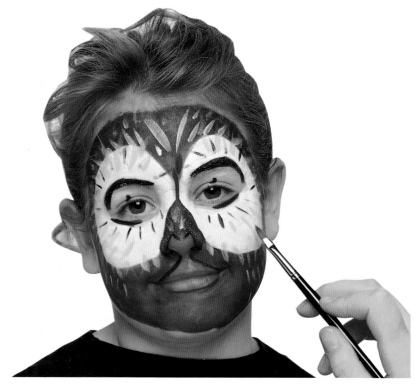

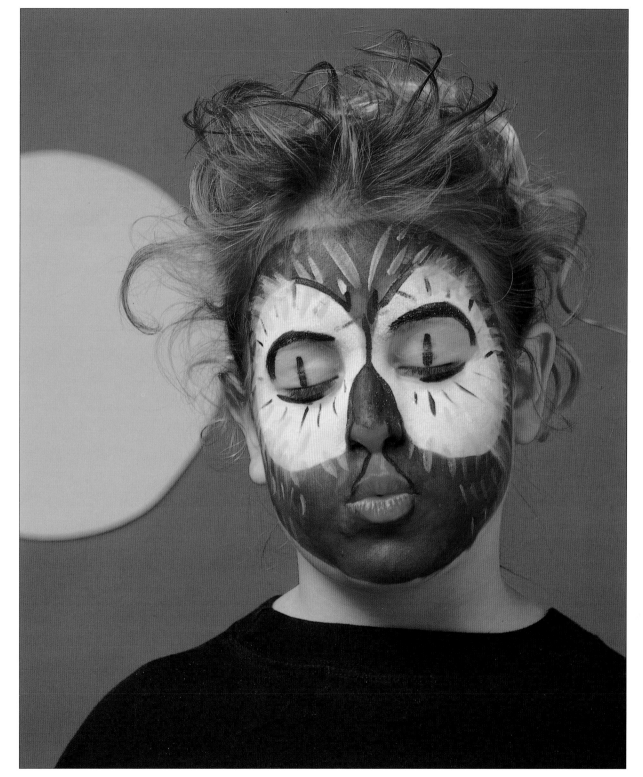

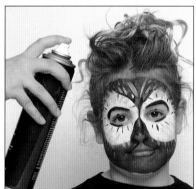

6 Brush the hair off the face into feathery tufts and secure it with hair spray and hair clips.

Monkey

For the complete monkey outfit make a pair of furry ears and wear brown clothes. You could even make a brown tail.

YOU WILL NEED
make-up sponge
water-based face paints
fine make-up brush
medium make-up brush

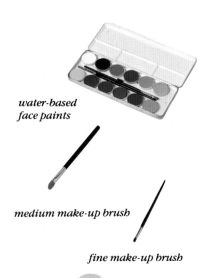

water-based face paints

medium make-up brush

fine make-up brush

make-up sponge

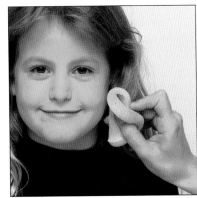

1 Using a damp sponge, apply a yellow base colour over the face.

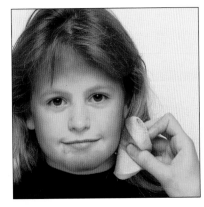

2 Rinse the sponge, then dab a few darker shades around the edge of the face, blending them in with the base.

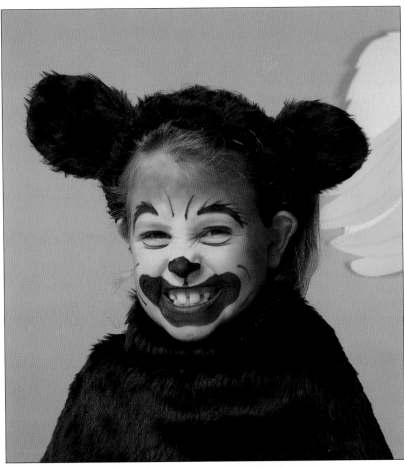

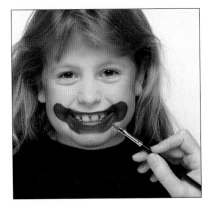

3 Paint the outline of the monkey's mouth using a fine brush. Use a medium brush to fill in the marked area with black.

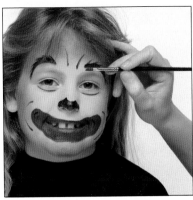

4 Paint the tip of the nose black and paint on a pair of eyebrows above the model's own. Using a fine brush, paint a few lines in between the eyebrows, under each eye and at each side of the mouth.

Panda

If you only have a few face paints, this is the perfect project for you. It is good for beginners as it is simple to do. Use the template and the instructions provided earlier to make a pair of furry ears to match.

YOU WILL NEED
black make-up (eye-liner) pencil
make-up sponge
water-based face paints
medium make-up brush
fine make-up brush

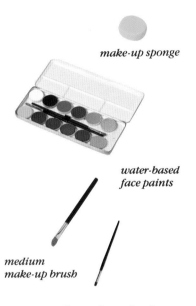

make-up sponge

water-based face paints

medium make-up brush

fine make-up brush

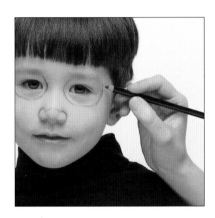

1 Using a black make-up (eye-liner) pencil, gently draw an outline around each eye as shown. Draw an outline across the tip of the nose.

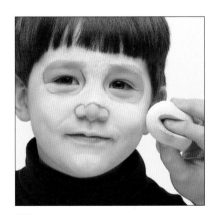

2 Using a damp sponge, apply a white base over the face, avoiding the areas you have just marked with the pencil.

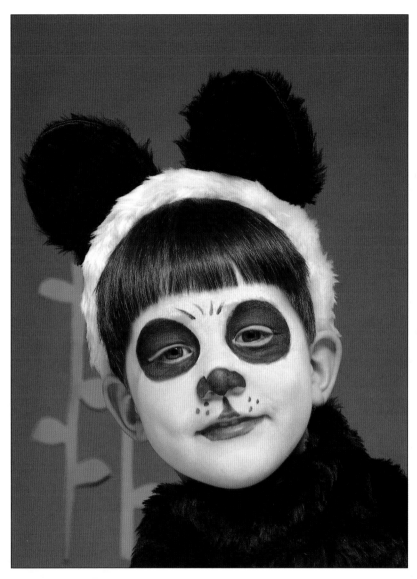

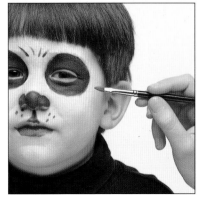

3 Using a medium brush, paint the eyes and the tip of the nose black. Using a fine brush, paint a line joining the nose to the mouth and paint the lips. Paint small whisker spots either side of the mouth. Add black lines between the eyebrows.

GHOULS, GHOSTS AND MONSTERS

Witch

This young witch looks like she's got a few tricks up her sleeve. She is wearing a cloak made from an old piece of fabric and long black nails.

YOU WILL NEED
tape measure
black fabric for hat
iron-on interfacing (optional)
pencil
scissors
needle and thread
raffia or straw

FOR THE FACE
make-up sponge
water-based face paints
lipstick brush
fine make-up brush
thick make-up brush

black fabric

thread

raffia

iron-on interfacing

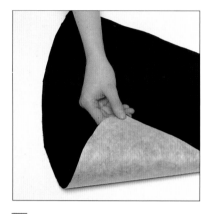

1 To make the hat, measure the width of your head so that you know how wide to make the rim of the hat. If the fabric you are using needs to be stiffened, iron a piece of interfacing onto the reverse side. Ask an adult to help you. Draw and cut out a triangle with a curved base, making sure the rim measures the width of your head with a small allowance for sewing the fabric together.

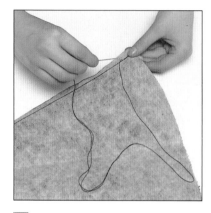

2 With the right sides facing, fold the triangle in half to form a tall cone and sew along the side.

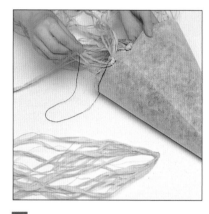

3 Make bundles of raffia or straw and tie a knot in the centre of each bundle. Sew each bundle around the rim of the hat leaving a gap at the front. The more bundles you sew on, the wilder the wig will be. Turn the hat the right way out.

scissors

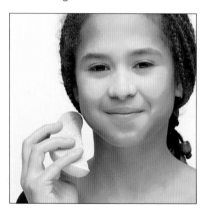

4 For the face, use a damp sponge to dab the base colours over the face.

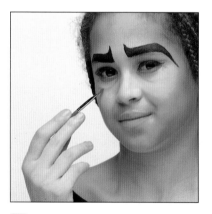

5 Using a lipstick brush, paint on a pair of wild, black eyebrows. Paint a black line on each eyelid just above the eyelashes. Paint a line of red just under each eye and a black curve below it.

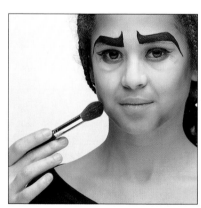

6 Add ageing lines with a fine brush Build more colour onto the cheeks using a thick make-up brush. Paint the lips red, exaggerating the top lip.

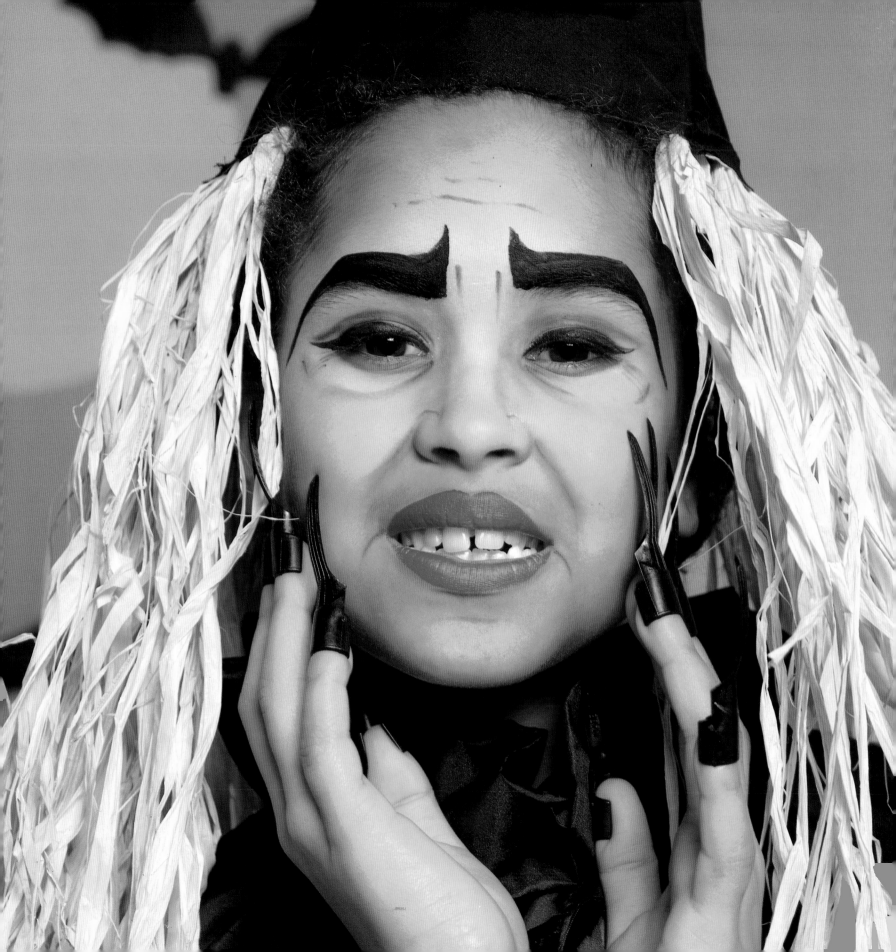

Ghost

Spook your friends in this fabulous disguise. See how long it takes before they guess who you are.

YOU WILL NEED
old white sheet
scissors
needle and thread or sewing machine
milliner's wire
black felt
fabric glue

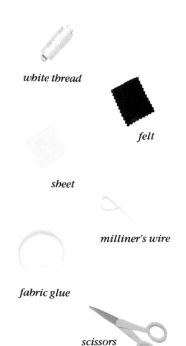

white thread

felt

sheet

milliner's wire

fabric glue

scissors

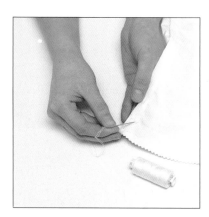

1 Cut two pieces of sheet in the shape of a dome, making sure the height of the dome is longer than you own height. Sew the two pieces together leaving an opening at the bottom. Sew another line of stitching parallel to the line you have sewn. This is to make a tube for the wire.

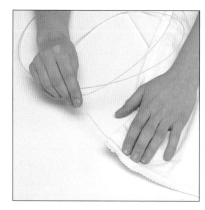

2 Thread the wire through the tube. Secure each end of the wire to the sheet with a few stitches.

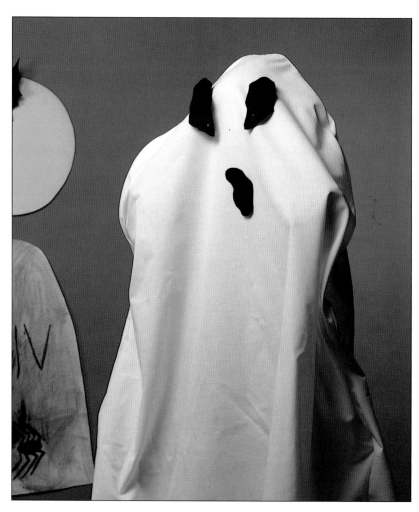

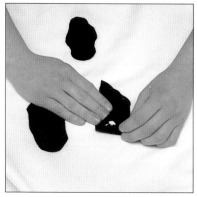

3 Cut out a mouth and pair of eyes from a piece of felt and glue them onto the sheet using fabric glue.

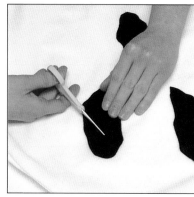

4 Cut small holes in the eyes and the mouth, so that you can see where you are going. Try the costume on and bend the wire to fit your body.

Egyptian Mummy

Make sure you wear a white T-shirt and a pair of white tights or leggings underneath the costume, just in case it starts to unravel!

YOU WILL NEED
old white sheet
scissors
needle and thread
white T-shirt and leggings or tights

FOR THE FACE
make-up sponge
water-based face paints

sheet

thread

scissors

water-based face paints

make-up sponge

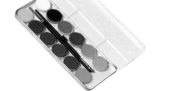

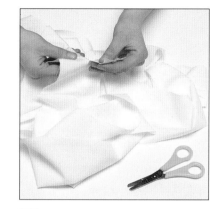

1 To make the costume, tear or cut strips of the sheet approximately 10 cm/4 in wide and as long as possible.

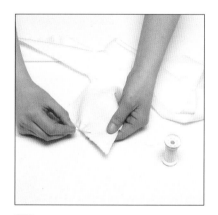

2 Sew the strips of fabric together to form one long strip.

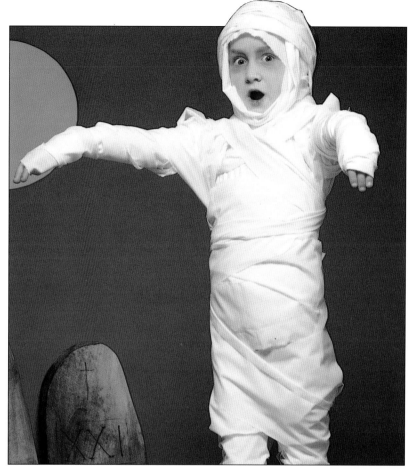

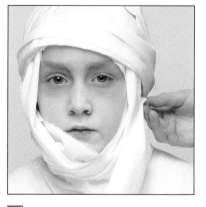

3 For the face, use a damp sponge to apply a white base. Rinse the sponge, then dab light purple around the eye sockets to give a ghoulish appearance. Then wrap the fabric round the head first, leaving the face open. Gradually wrap the fabric down the body.

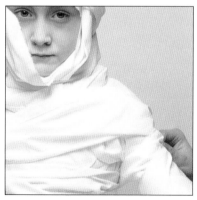

4 When you get to the hands, go back up the arm again, still wrapping the fabric around. Do the same with the legs. When you have wrapped the whole body, sew the end of the strip to part of the costume. To take the costume off, simply unravel the strip of fabric.

Vampire

Dress all in black for this costume. Don't be surprised if you frighten your friends and family with your haunted face.

YOU WILL NEED
make-up sponge
water-based face paints
medium make-up brush
fine make-up brush
black make-up (eyeliner) pencil
  (optional)
red make-up (eyeliner) pencil
fake blood (optional)

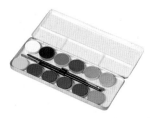

water-based face paints

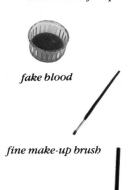

fake blood

fine make-up brush

medium make-up brush

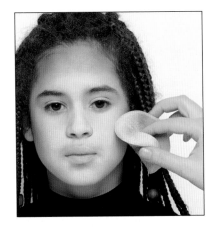

1 Using a damp sponge, apply a base colour on the face. Rinse the sponge, then dab a slightly darker shade on the forehead, blending it with the base colour.

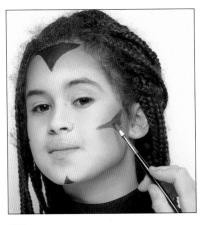

2 Using a medium brush, paint a triangle in the centre of the forehead, one on either side of the face at the cheekbones and a small one at the bottom of the chin. You might find it easier to draw the outline for each shape first, to make sure they are symmetrical, and then fill them in.

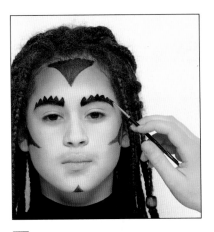

3 Using a fine brush paint a pair of jagged eyebrows over the model's own. Again, you may find it easier to draw the outline first.

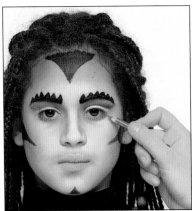

4 Paint the eyelids white and the area up to the eyebrows grey. Use the red make-up pencil to colour the area under the eyes .

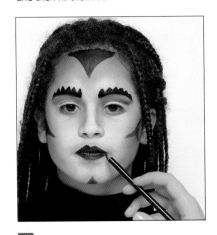

5 Exaggerate the points on the top lip and colour the lips black.

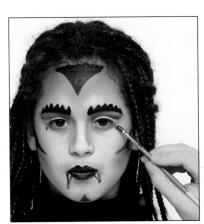

6 Paint the outline of long, pointed fangs under the bottom lip and fill them in with yellow. Dab fake blood or red make-up at the points of the fangs and at the corners of the eyes

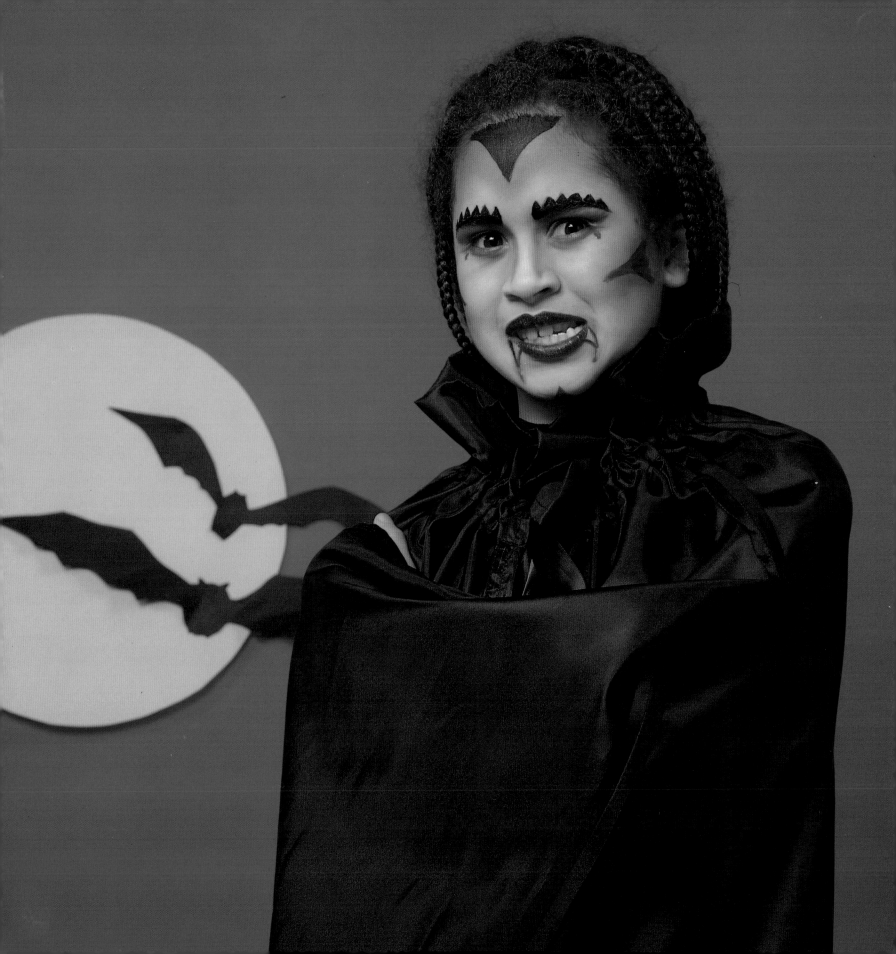

Martian

Try decorating an old pair of tights or leggings in a similar style to the T-shirt and give an old pair of shoes a "space lift" with paint and glitter.

YOU WILL NEED
4 paper baubles (balls)
hairband
paints
paintbrush
glue
glitter
glitter glue
sequins
ribbon or elastic
T-shirt
felt
scissors
fabric glue
fabric paints

FOR THE FACE
make-up sponge
water-based face paints
stipple sponge
medium make-up brush
glitter gel
lipstick brush

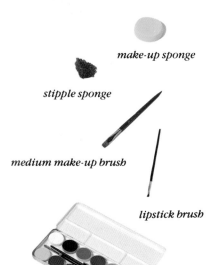

make-up sponge

stipple sponge

medium make-up brush

lipstick brush

water-based face paints

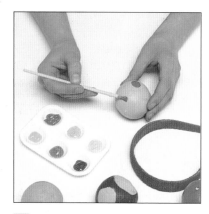

1 To make the costume, paint the baubles (balls) and the hairband and leave them to dry. Using contrasting colours, paint spots on the baubles.

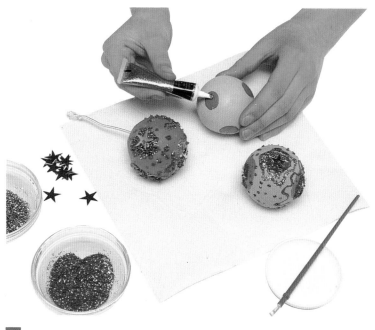

2 Paint areas of the baubles with glue and dip them into the glitter. Use glitter glue to make exciting shapes and patterns and glue on a few sequins. Try to create a different pattern on each bauble.

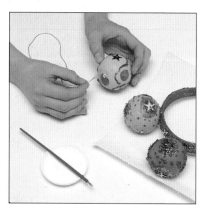

3 Glue three baubles onto the hairband. For the necklace, glue the two ends of the ribbon or elastic into a small hole on the fourth bauble. Allow the glue to dry before trying on the accessories.

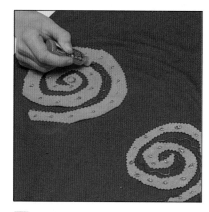

4 To decorate the T-shirt, cut out two spiral shapes from coloured felt and using fabric glue, stick them onto the T-shirt. Decorate the spirals with fabric paints and glitter glue.

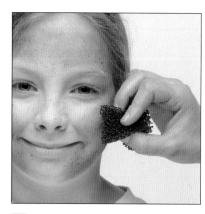

5 For the face, use a damp sponge to apply the base colour. Using a stipple sponge, dab a slightly darker shade over the base colour to add texture.

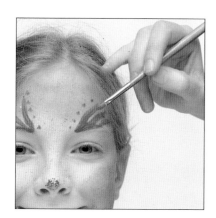

6 Using a medium brush, paint on a pair of wiggly eyebrows as shown. Using glitter gel in a contrasting colour, paint a spot on the tip of the nose.

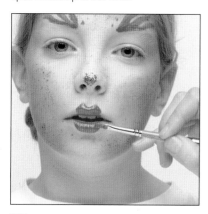

7 Using a lipstick brush, paint a tiny mouth as shown, avoiding the corners of the mouth.

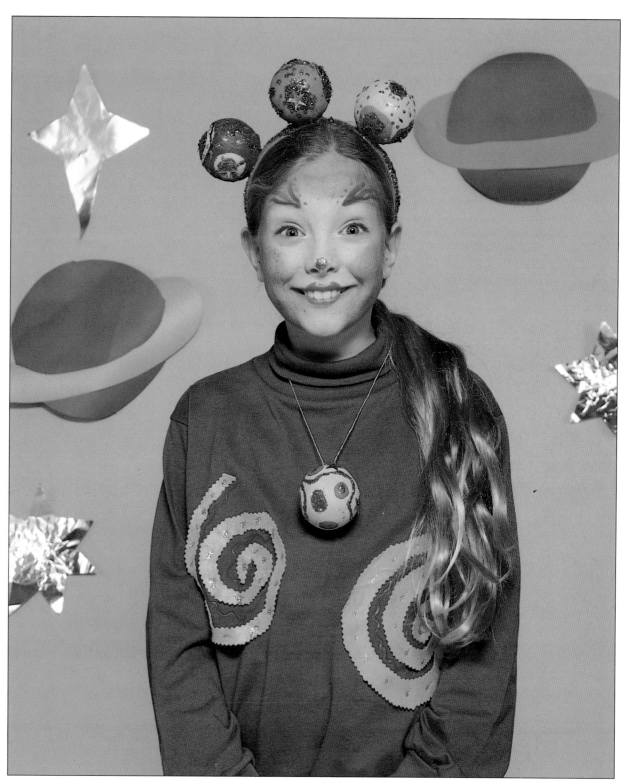

Frankenstein's Monster

Practise your monster's walk when you wear this costume. This will really scare your friends.

YOU WILL NEED
make-up sponge
water-based face paints
thick make-up brush
medium make-up brush
fine make-up brush
black swimming hat (bathing cap)

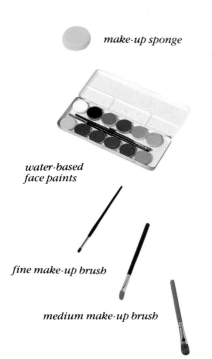

make-up sponge

water-based face paints

fine make-up brush

medium make-up brush

thick make-up brush

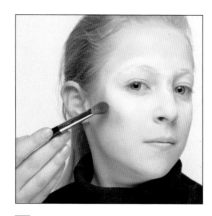

1 Using a damp sponge, apply the base colour over the face. Rinse the sponge, then apply a darker shade, avoiding the mouth and the nose area. Finally, shade the cheekbones with a third colour.

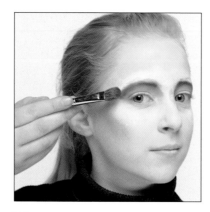

2 Using a medium brush, paint the eyebrows black and darken the eyelids and the area under each eye.

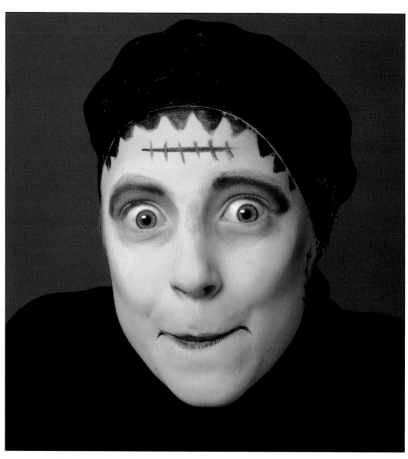

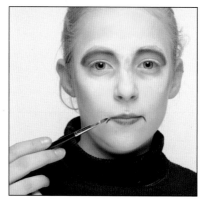

3 Paint the lips black and, using a fine brush, paint fine black lines at either side of the mouth.

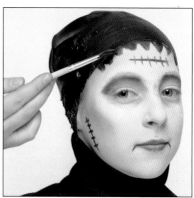

4 Using a fine brush, paint a black scar on the forehead and on one side of the face. Put on a black swimming hat (bathing cap), making sure you hide most of the hair. Where the hat meets the forehead paint a jagged hair line.

Purple Monster

If you want to be a really gruesome monster, wear a set of rotten-looking plastic teeth. They can be bought from toy or joke shops.

YOU WILL NEED
make-up sponge
water-based face paints
fine make-up brush
medium make-up brush

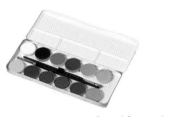

water-based face paints

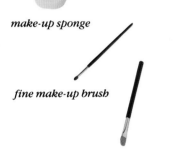

make-up sponge

fine make-up brush

medium make-up brush

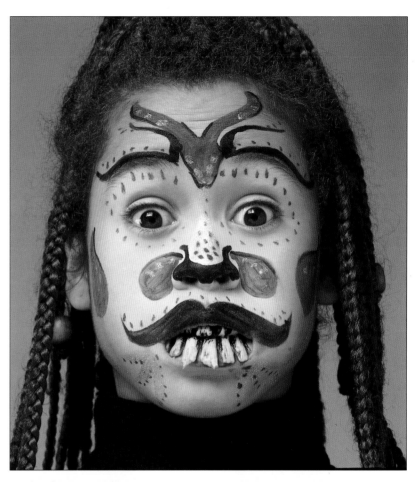

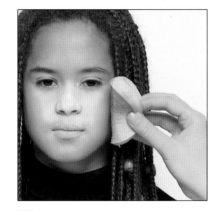

1 Using a damp sponge, apply the base colour over the face. Dab a darker shade around the edge of the face and on the forehead, blending it with the base colour.

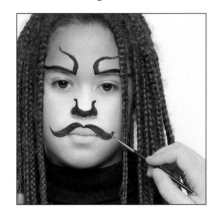

2 Using a fine brush, paint a pair of eyebrows slightly above the model's own. Paint the tip of the nose and paint on a droopy moustache just above the model's mouth. You might find it easier to sketch an outline for the shapes first and then fill them in.

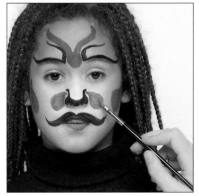

3 Use a medium brush to paint on other shapes. Paint the shapes on one side of the face first and then paint the other side. This will help you to make sure the design is symmetrical. Paint the lips the same colour.

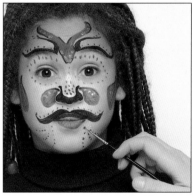

4 Decorate the face with silver and purple spots and other details.

Skeleton

This is the perfect outfit for spooking your friends and family on Hallowe'en.

YOU WILL NEED
black leotard
white fabric paints
paintbrush
black leggings

FOR THE FACE
black make-up (eye-liner) pencil
water-based face paints
medium make-up brush

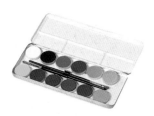

water-based face paints

medium make-up brush

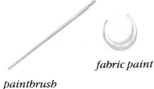

fabric paint

paintbrush

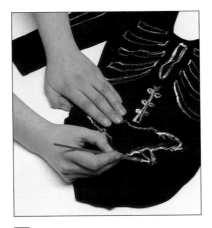

1 To make the costume, use fabric paints to draw on the outline of the skeleton's body, making sure the leotard is lying flat.

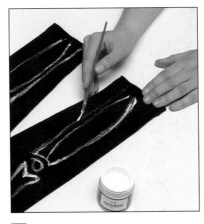

2 Paint the outline of the skeleton's legs on the front of the leggings.

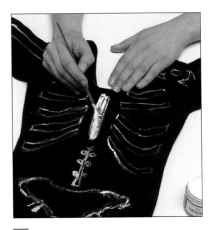

3 Fill in the outlined areas with white on both the leotard and leggings.

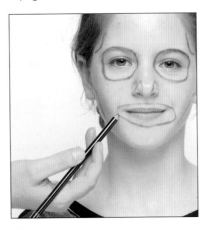

4 Using a black make-up (eye-liner) pencil, draw a circular outline around each eye, a small triangle above each nostril, and a large mouth shape around the model's own mouth. Draw an outline around the edge of the face.

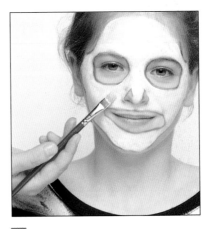

5 Using a medium brush, paint the face white, avoiding the shapes you have just drawn in pencil.

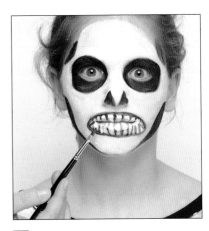

6 Paint the eyes, the triangles above the nostrils and the sides of the face black. Paint a thick black outline around the mouth and fill the mouth area in white. Divide the mouth into a set of ghostly teeth with black lines.

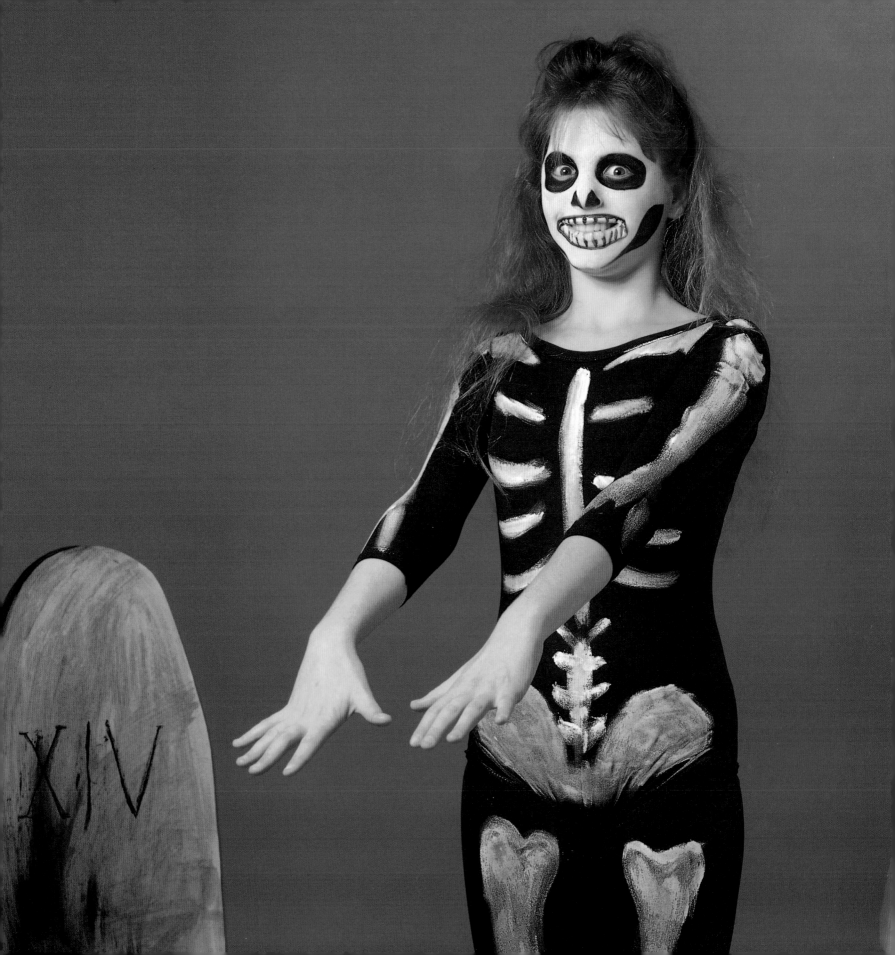

XIV

Zombie

You could dress in black to make this character look even more creepy.

YOU WILL NEED
make-up sponge
water-based face paints
thick make-up brush
medium make-up brush
fine make-up brush
fake blood (optional)

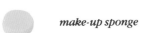

make-up sponge

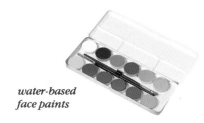

*water-based
face paints*

fine make-up brush

thick make-up brush

*medium
make-up brush*

fake blood

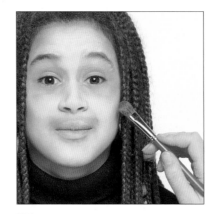

1 Using a damp sponge, apply the base colour over the face, avoiding the area surrounding the eye. Use a thick brush to dust a darker colour on the forehead, around each eye and around the mouth, to create a bruised effect.

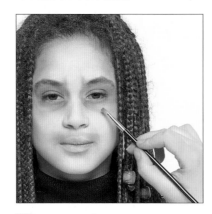

2 Using a medium brush, fill in the area surrounding the eye with a darker colour, then paint dark lines under the eyes and on the eyebrows.

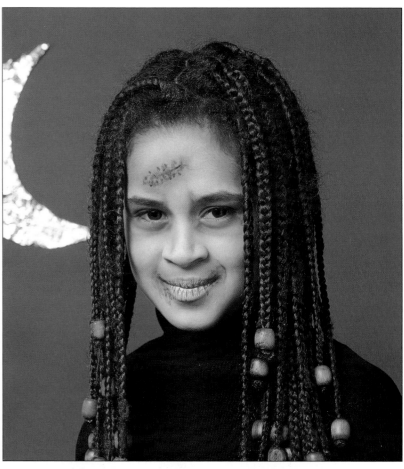

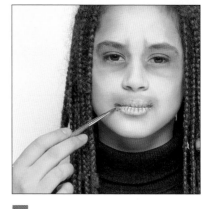

3 Paint the lips a light colour and use a fine brush to paint on dark lines, making the lips look as if they are cracked. Using fake blood or red make-up, paint the corners of the mouth to look as if they are bleeding.

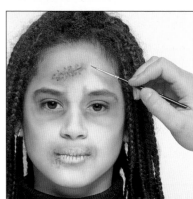

4 Use a fine brush to paint the scar on the forehead.

Gremlin

This mischievous creature is all dressed in green.
Cover a green T-shirt with a piece of fur and wear a
pair of green tights.

YOU WILL NEED
tape measure
hairband
fake fur
scissors
needle and thread
glue
felt
template for ears
pencil

FOR THE FACE
water-based face paints
medium make-up brush

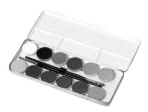

water-based face paints

medium make-up brush

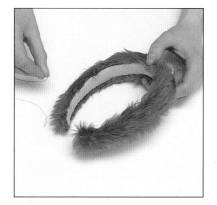

1 Measure the length of the hairband
and cut the fake fur to fit. Sew the fur
onto the hairband, then sew or glue a
strip of felt to the inside.

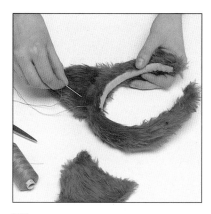

2 Using the template, draw and cut out
two pieces of fur for each ear. With right
sides facing, sew the two ear pieces
together. Turn right side out and stitch
onto the hairband.

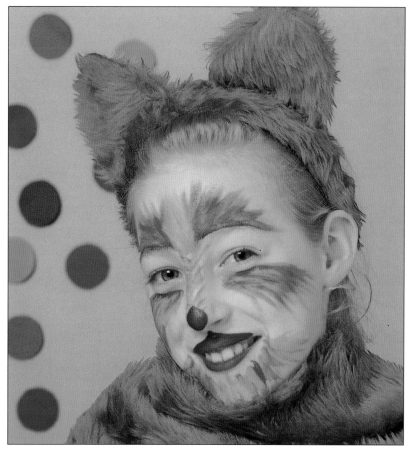

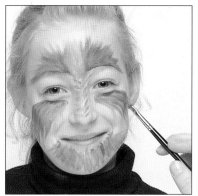

3 For the face, apply green areas with
feathery brush strokes.

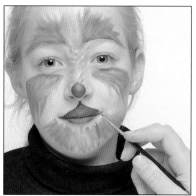

4 Paint a brown spot at the end of the
nose and paint the lips the same colour,
enlarging the top lip so that it meets the
tip of the nose.

Dinosaur

Dress up as a prehistoric monster in this spiky camouflaged outfit.

YOU WILL NEED
**green fabric or felt
scissors
green polo neck (turtleneck) or
    T-shirt
fabric glue
needle and thread
fire resistant stuffing (batting)
hairband
green paint
paintbrush
glue**

FOR THE FACE
**make-up sponge
water-based face paints
stipple sponge
medium make-up brush**

hairband

thread

fabric

fabric glue

stuffing (batting)

scissors

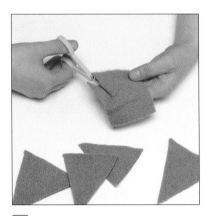

1 To make the costume, cut out lots of triangles, more or less the same size, from a piece of old green fabric or felt. You could use different coloured green fabrics if you don't have enough of one kind.

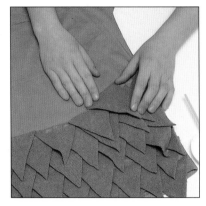

2 Starting at the bottom of the shirt, glue on the fabric spikes so that they overlap each other. Leave a circle in the centre of the shirt empty.

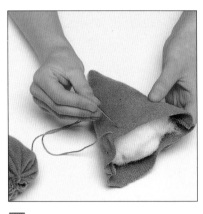

3 For each spike on the spine, you will need to cut out two triangles. Sew the two triangles together with right sides facing. Turn the triangles right side out and fill with stuffing (batting) to make a spike shape. Sew a running stitch around the bottom edge of the spike and pull gently. This will draw up the threads and close the spike. Tie a knot.

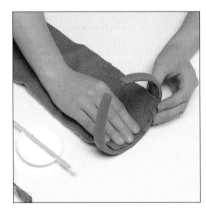

4 Paint the hairband green and leave it to dry. Cut a strip of green fabric approximately 10 cm/4 in wide and however long you wish it to be. Using glue, secure the strip onto the inside of the hairband and leave to dry.

5 Sew the spikes onto the strip of fabric attached to the hairband.

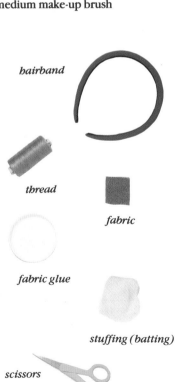

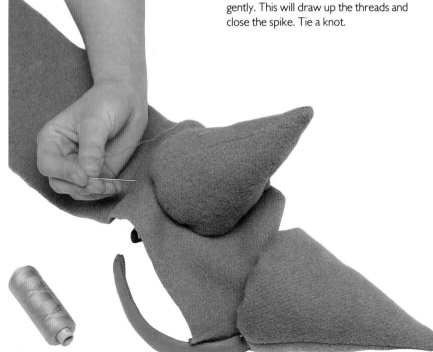

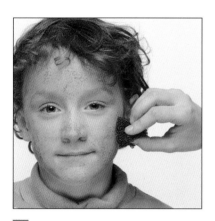

6 For the face, use a damp sponge to apply the base colour over the face. Using a stipple sponge, dab a darker shade over the base colour.

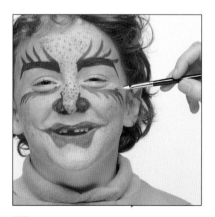

7 Using a medium brush, decorate the face. Paint on wild eyebrows, exaggerated nostrils, spots, big lips and markings under each eye.

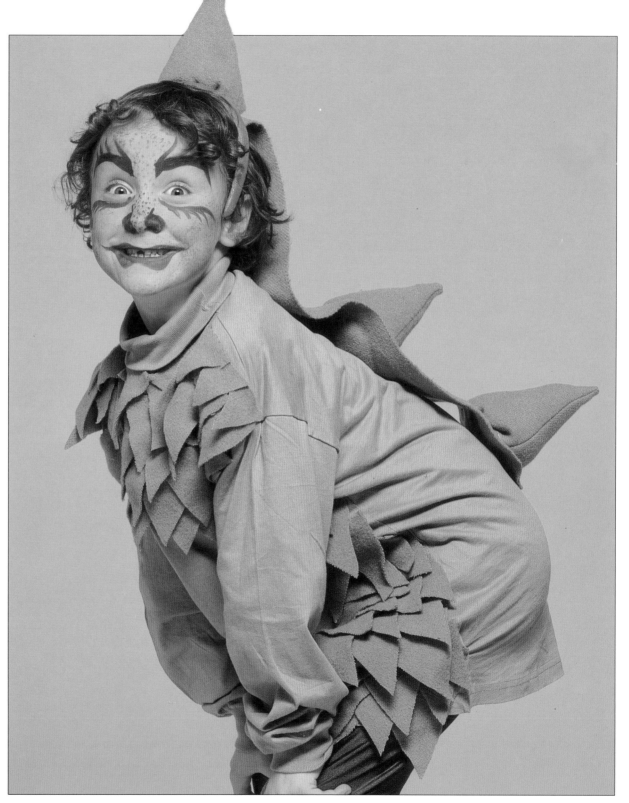

FUN AND FANTASY FIGURES

Clown

Bounce around in this jolly outfit and entertain your friends and family. Decorate a hat and an old pair of shoes to match the colourful costume.

YOU WILL NEED
6 self-covering buttons
scraps of fabric
template for clown button
pencil
coloured felt
scissors
needle and thread
old shirt
old pair of trousers (pants)
fabric glue
milliner's wire
broad ribbon
fabric for the bow tie
narrow ribbon

FOR THE FACE
make-up sponge
water-based face paints
black make-up (eye-liner) pencil
medium make-up brush
fine make-up brush
thick make-up brush

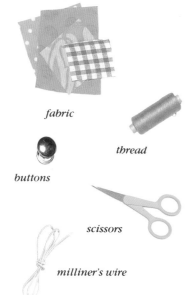

fabric

thread

buttons

scissors

milliner's wire

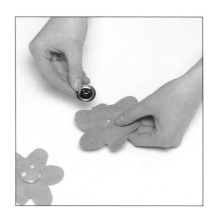

1 To make the costume, cover each button in a different scrap of fabric. Using the template, draw and cut out a flower shape from a piece of felt and snip a hole in the centre of it. Fix the flower onto the back of the button and secure on the back. Sew the buttons onto the shirt and trousers (pants).

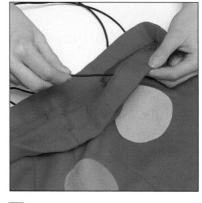

2 Cut out large dots of felt and stick them onto the trousers with fabric glue. Thread a piece of milliner's wire through the waistband. Twist the two ends of the wire together to secure them.

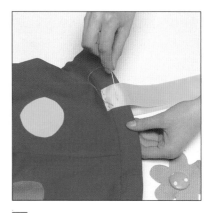

3 Sew two separate lengths of ribbon onto the waist of the trousers to make a pair of braces (suspenders). Sew a covered button onto each brace.

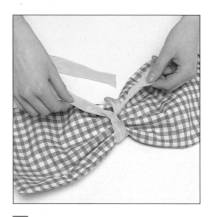

4 To make the bow tie, sew two rectangular pieces of fabric together with the right sides facing, leaving a gap. Turn right side out and stitch the gap. Tie a piece of ribbon around the centre of the rectangle and tie a knot. Tie around the clown's neck under the shirt collar.

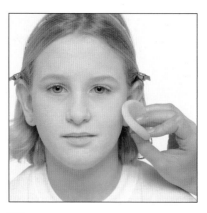

5 For the face, use a damp sponge to apply a smooth white base.

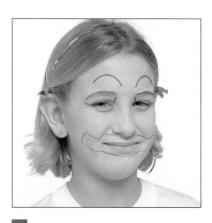

6 Using a black make-up (eye-liner) pencil, draw the outline of a clown's mouth. Draw a pair of eyebrows above the model's own and gently mark an area around each eye as shown.

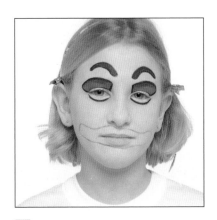

7 Using a medium brush, paint the area around each eye with lots of colour and paint over the drawn eyebrows with a thick black line.

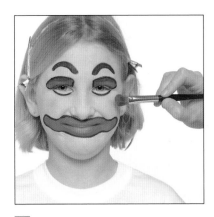

8 Using a fine brush, paint the mouth red, and outline the shape of the mouth in black. Using a thick brush, colour the cheeks a rosy red.

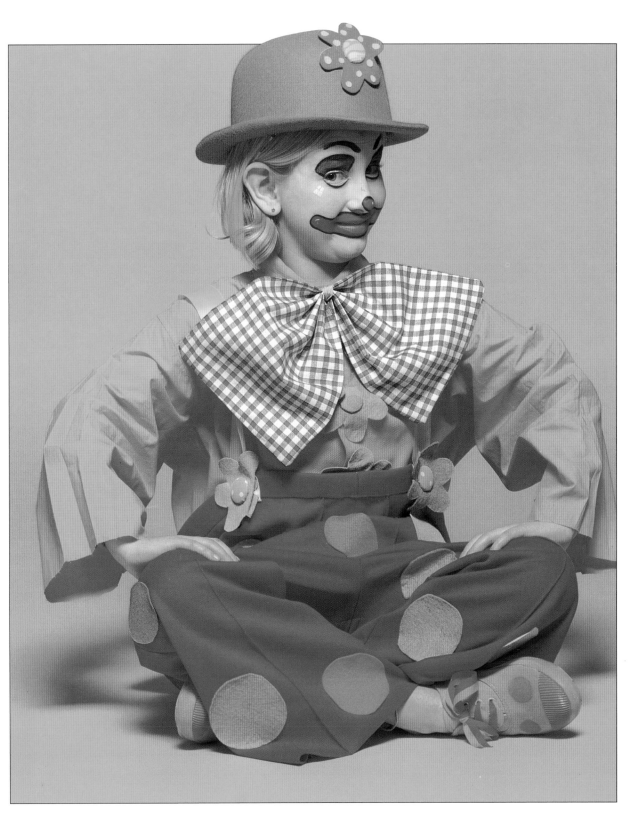

Ballerina

Show off your ballet steps in this pretty tutu. Make it the same colour as your ballet leotard.

YOU WILL NEED
2 metres/2 yards coloured netting
needle, thread and pins
tape measure
wide ribbon for the waistband
narrow ribbon for the bows
scissors
matching leotard and tights

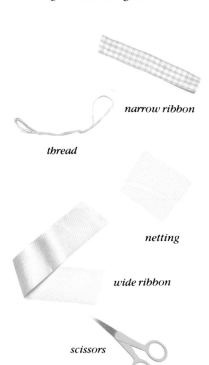

narrow ribbon

thread

netting

wide ribbon

scissors

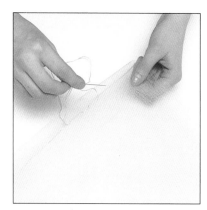

1 Fold the netting over lengthwise and sew a line of running stitch along the folded edge. Measure your ballerina's waist. For a short tutu, fold over again, and secure with running stitches. Pull the thread gently to gather the netting to fit the waist and tie a knot or sew a few stitches to secure the gathers.

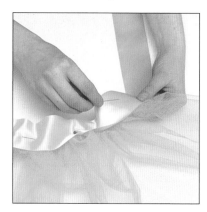

2 Pin the wide ribbon onto the gathered netting and then sew it on.

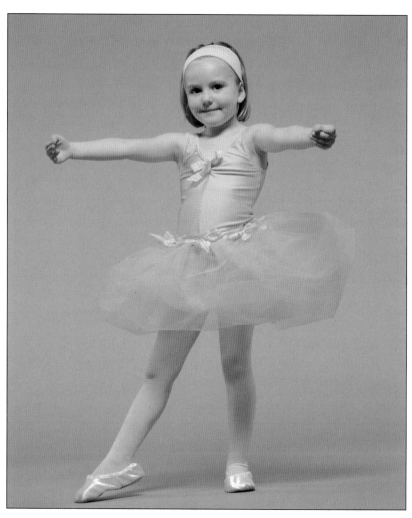

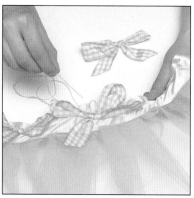

3 Using the narrower ribbon, tie approximately six small bows. Sew five bows onto the waistband.

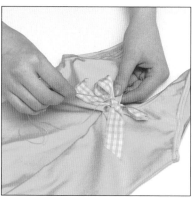

4 To finish the costume, sew the last bow onto the leotard.

Fairy

Dress up in this sparkling outfit and make a special wish. For a magical effect, wear a white leotard and pin some tinsel in your hair.

YOU WILL NEED
2 metres/2 yards netting
needle and thread
scissors
tinsel
1.5 metres/1½ yards white fabric
milliner's wire
silver elastic cord
garden cane
silver paint
paintbrush
silver paper or cardboard
adhesive tape
glue
white leotard and tights

paintbrush

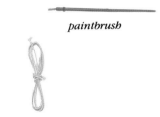

milliner's wire

garden cane   *fabric*

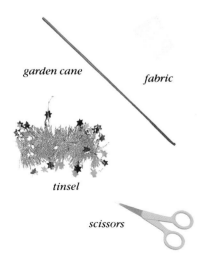

tinsel

scissors

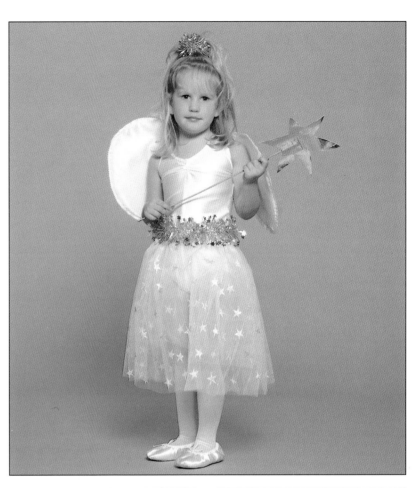

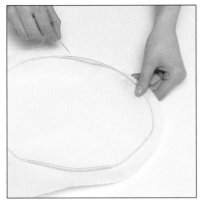

1 To make the tutu, follow the instructions for the ballerina tutu, folding the netting lengthwise once only for a longer skirt. Instead of decorating the waistband with ribbon, sew on a piece of tinsel. Cut out two pieces of white fabric for the wings, in a figure-of-eight shape. On the wrong side of one of the pieces of fabric, sew a separate length of wire around each wing.

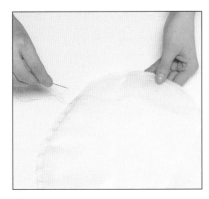

2 Place the other piece of fabric on top of the first, making sure the wrong sides are facing. Sew around the edge to secure the two pieces together.

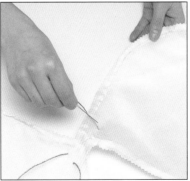

3 Sew a loop of elastic cord onto each wing, near the centre. These will slip over the arms to support the wings on the body.

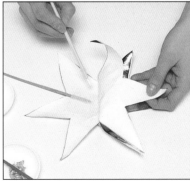

4 To make the wand, first paint a garden cane silver and leave it to dry. Cut out two silver stars and fasten the silver stick onto the reverse side of one of the stars with a piece of adhesive tape. Glue the stars together.

Scarecrow

If you don't have any suitable old clothes of your own, visit a second-hand clothes shop or rummage through piles of clothes at a local flea market. The older the clothes are the better the costume will be.

YOU WILL NEED
raffia
old felt hat
scissors
plastic toy mouse
glue
needle and thread
old clothes, such as a jacket and
    trousers (pants)
scraps of fabric
orange cardboard
orange paint
paintbrush
elastic cord

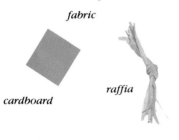
fabric

cardboard   *raffia*

scissors

paint

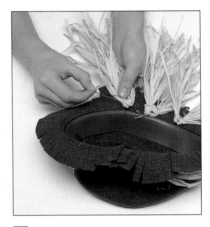

1 Tie a few strands of raffia around the hat. Cut a fringe into the rim of the hat with a pair of scissors. Glue a plastic mouse on the top of the hat.

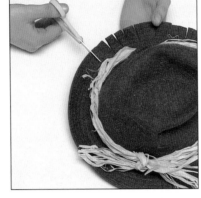

2 Tie bundles of raffia in a knot and sew the bundles around the inside rim of the hat, leaving a gap at the front.

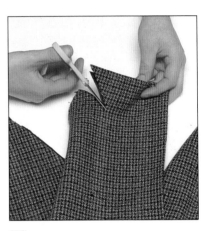

3 Cut ragged edges on the jacket and the trousers (pants).

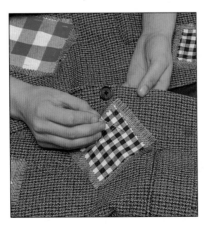

4 Cut scraps of fabric into squares and rectangles and sew them onto the jacket and the trousers.

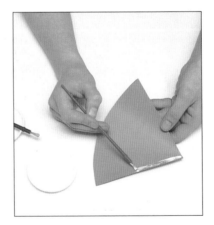

5 To make the nose, cut a piece of orange cardboard into a cone shape. Roll the cardboard into a cone and glue it together.

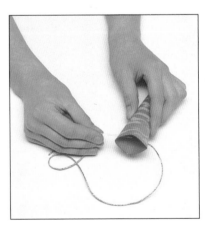

6 Paint orange lines around the cone and leave them to dry. Make a small hole on either side of the cone and thread a piece of elastic cord through that will fit around your head. Tie a knot at each end of the elastic.

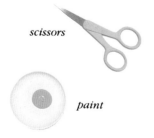

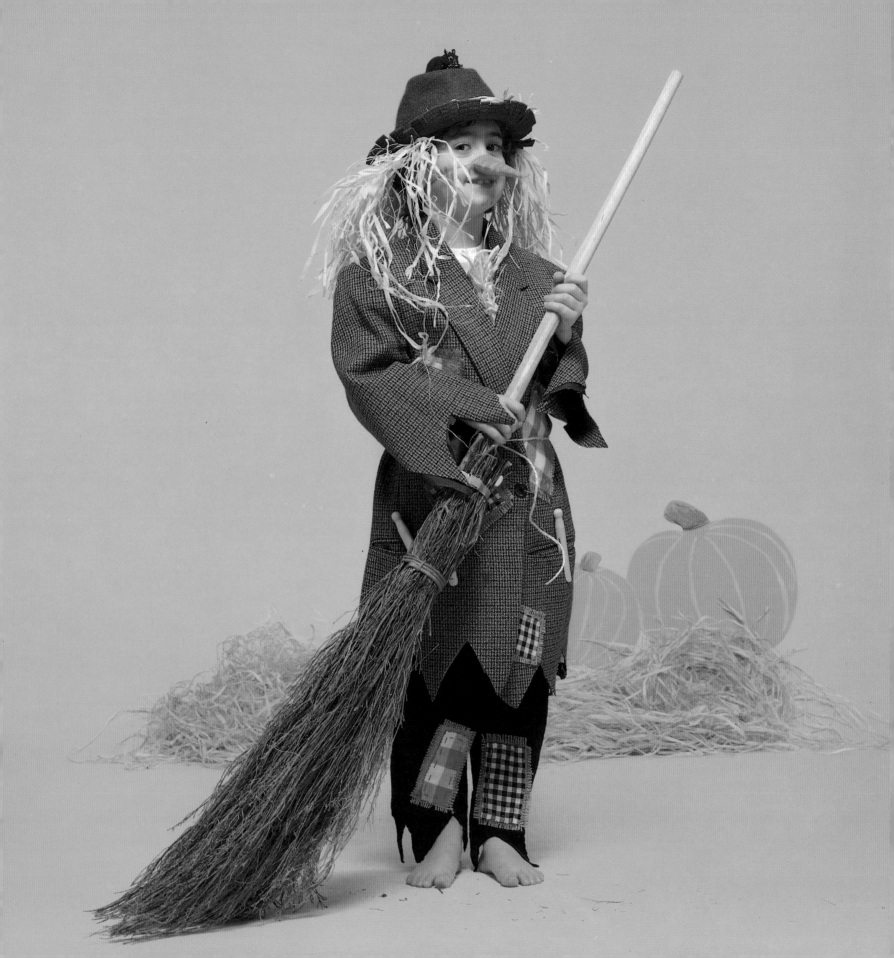

Angel

To make the tutu, follow the instructions for the ballerina, but sew a piece of tinsel onto the waistband instead of the ribbon. Make the wings the same way as for the fairy costume.

YOU WILL NEED
hairband
2 paper baubles (balls)
silver paint
paintbrush
milliner's wire
tinsel
glue
white leotard and tights

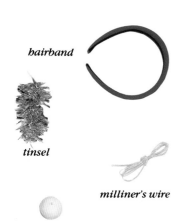

tinsel

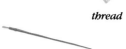

hairband

milliner's wire

paper bauble (ball)

thread

paintbrush

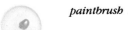

paint

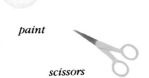

scissors

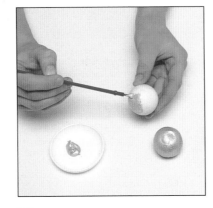

1 For the halo, paint the hairband and the two paper baubles (balls) silver and leave them to dry.

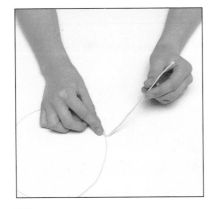

2 Bend a piece of milliner's wire in a circle and twist the ends together to secure them. Attach two separate lengths of wire approximately 7.5 cm/3 in long to the wire circle.

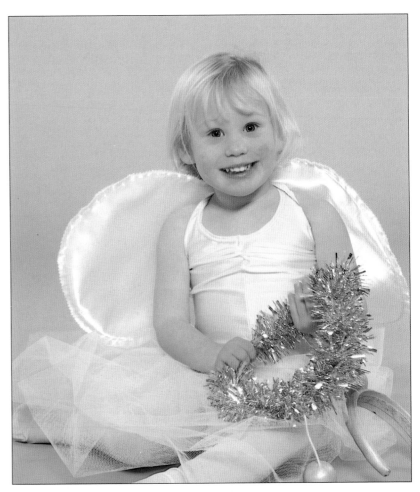

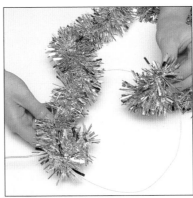

3 Wrap a piece of tinsel around the wire circle.

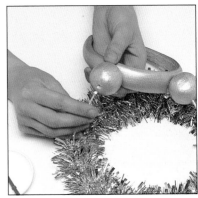

4 Glue the silver baubles onto the hairband and leave the glue to harden. Make a small hole in each bauble and fix the ends of the wire into the holes with a little glue.

Devil

Make the devil a tail using an old red sock or one leg from a pair of tights. You could complete the costume with a trident and a set of false nails bought from a novelty shop.

YOU WILL NEED
hairband
tape measure
scissors
red felt
needle and thread
template for devil horns
pencil
thick interfacing

FOR THE FACE
make-up sponge
water-based face paints
fine make-up brush
medium make-up brush
lipstick brush

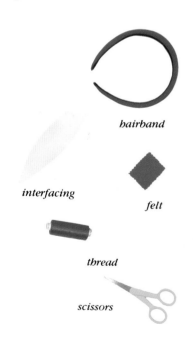

hairband

interfacing

felt

thread

scissors

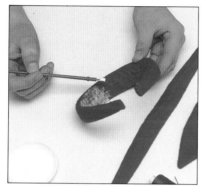

1 Make the ears as described in the animals chapter, covering the hairband with red felt and using the template for the devil horns. Place the two pieces of felt together with right sides facing and sew round the edges, leaving a gap to turn the right sides out. Do the same to the other ear. Cut a piece of interfacing to fit inside each ear; this will help to support them. Sew the ears onto the hairband.

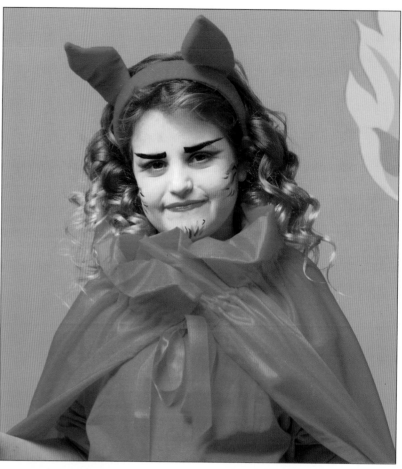

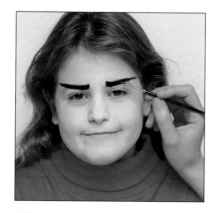

2 For the face, use a damp sponge to apply a smooth white base. Use a fine brush to paint a pair of eyebrows on top of the model's own.

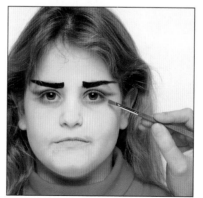

3 Using a medium brush, paint the eyelids a dark colour and paint the area under the eyes red. Using a lipstick brush, paint the lips red.

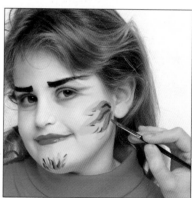

4 Paint a fiery flame on the model's chin and paint a similar design on the side of each cheek.

Robot

The fun part of this project is collecting all the bits and pieces to recycle. Ask your friends and family to help you collect interesting boxes, cartons and packages.

YOU WILL NEED
2 cardboard boxes
pencil
scissors
silver spray paint
cartons and containers made of
   cardboard and clear plastic
glue
3 Christmas baubles (balls)
foil pie-dishes (pans)
masking tape
pair of old shoes
2 metal kitchen scourers
tin foil

foil pie-dish
(pan)

Christmas
bauble (ball)

metal kitchen
scourer

egg carton

glue

silver spray

scissors

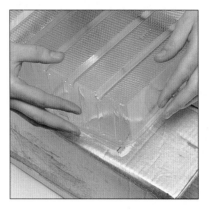

1 To make the helmet you will need a cardboard box that fits comfortably over your head. Draw a square on one side of the box and cut it out.

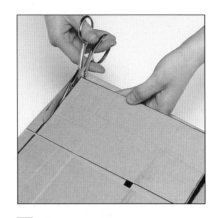

2 Ask an adult to help spray the box silver. You should do this outdoors or in a very airy room where the surfaces are well covered and protected. When the paint has dried, glue a clear plastic carton over the square hole. Punch a few holes in the carton to let air through.

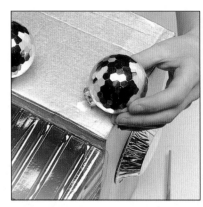

3 Decorate the box by gluing on Christmas baubles (balls) and foil pie-dishes (pans).

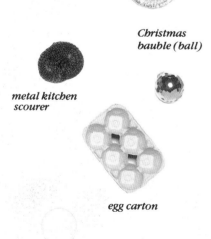

4 For the body of the robot, you will need a large cardboard box. Draw and cut out a hole on the top of the box for your head and one on either side for your arms. Secure the edges of the holes with masking tape.

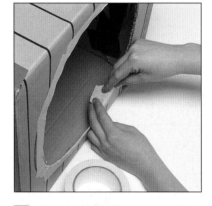

5 Decorate the robot body by gluing on all the boxes and containers you have been collecting. When the glue has dried, spray the box silver, following the same instructions as in step 2. Leave the paint to dry thoroughly before you try on the costume.

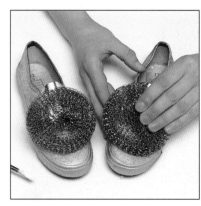

6 Spray a pair of old shoes silver and decorate them with a metal kitchen scourer or anything shiny. Finally, when you are dressed in your costume, ask a friend to wrap your arms and legs in tin foil to finish.

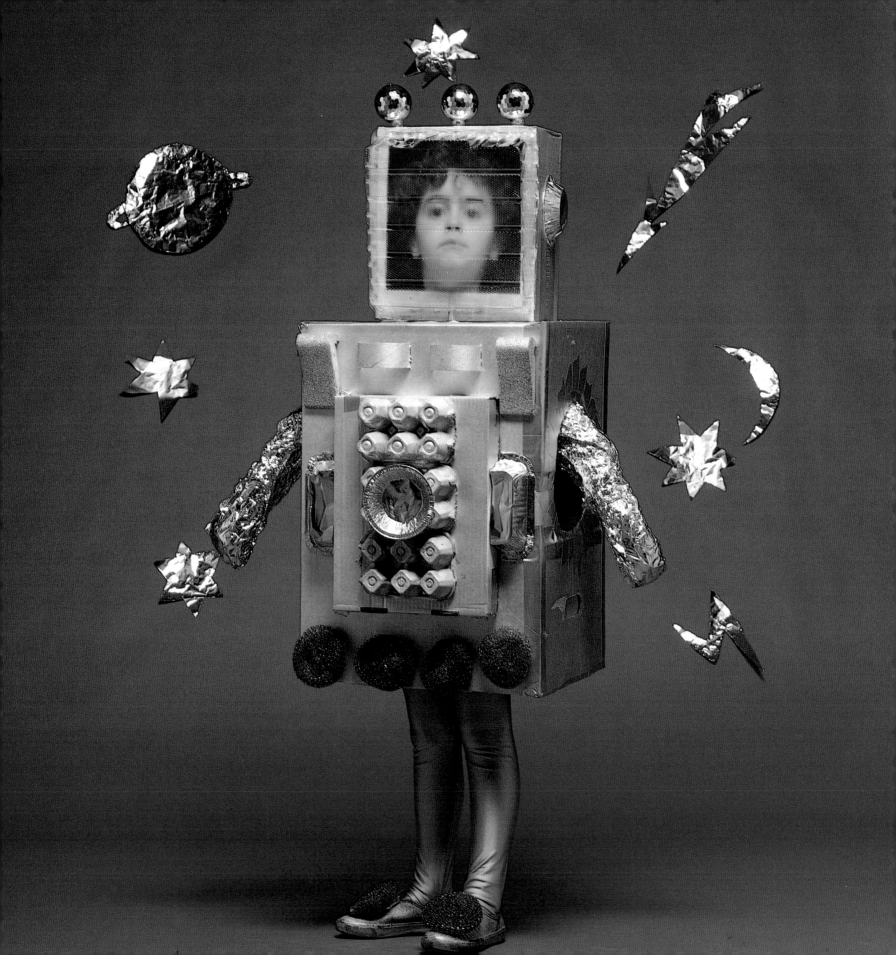

Astronaut

This space traveller looks all set for a journey to the stars and planets. Collect recycled containers to decorate the costume.

YOU WILL NEED
large balloon
PVA (white) glue
bowl
water
newspaper
pencil
scissors
silver paint
paintbrush
foil pie-dishes (pans)
tin foil
adhesive tape
piece of foam rubber
plain T-shirt
cardboard containers, such as fruit
    cartons
old pair of gloves (optional)

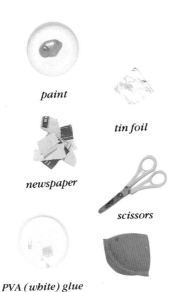

paint

newspaper

tin foil

scissors

PVA (white) glue

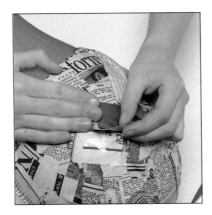

1 To make the helmet, blow up a large balloon and cover it with approximately 10 layers of papier mâché as described in the introduction. Leave to dry.

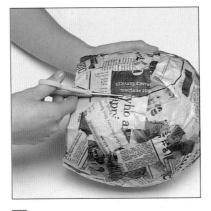

2 When the papier mâché has dried, pop the balloon with a pin. Draw and cut out an opening for the face and remove the balloon.

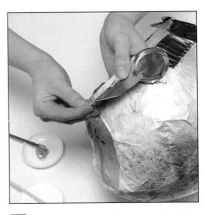

3 Paint the helmet silver and decorate with shapes cut from pie-dishes (pans).

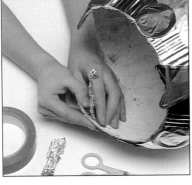

4 Make a microphone from a piece of rolled tin foil and tape it to the inside of the helmet. To make the helmet more comfortable to wear, glue a piece of foam rubber to the inside.

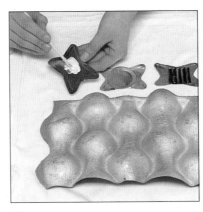

5 Decorate a plain T-shirt by gluing on containers and foil pie-dishes.

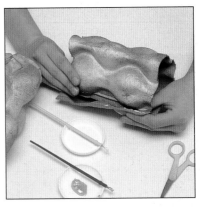

6 Make the arm and leg shields from cardboard containers. Fruit cartons have been used here. Paint the cartons silver and bend them to make a tube. Glue the edges together. If you have an old pair of gloves, paint them silver.

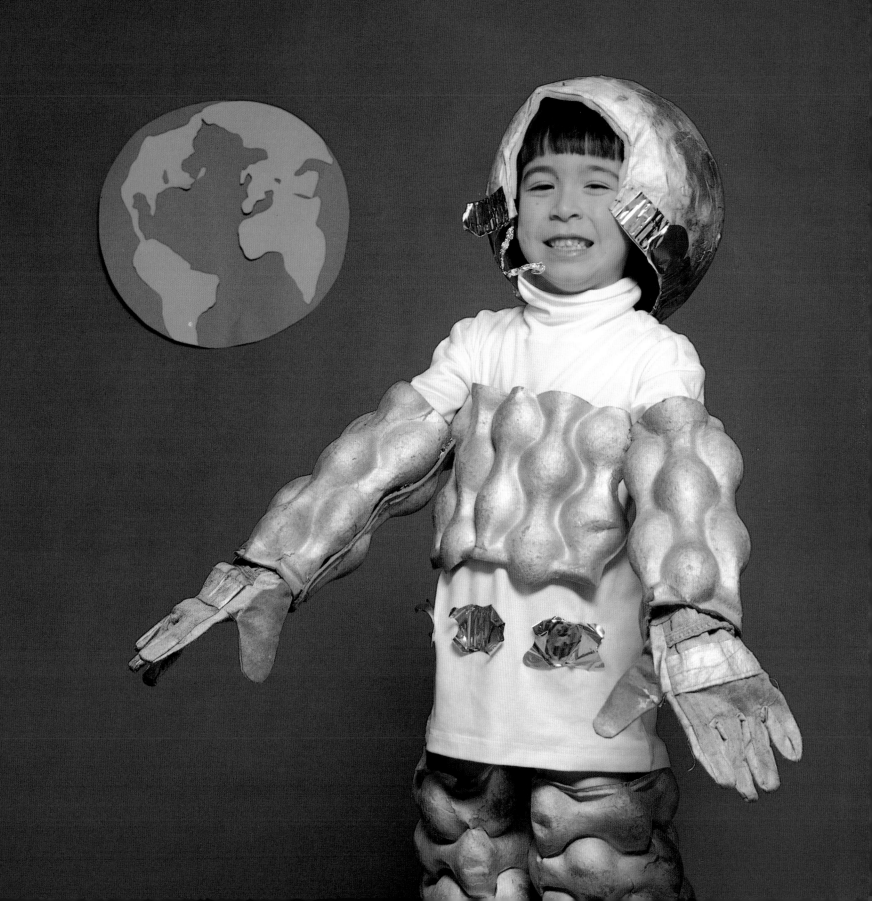

Sunflower

Dazzle your friends with this bright cheerful headdress. Wear yellow and green clothes to complete the costume.

YOU WILL NEED
pair of compasses
cardboard
scissors
ribbon
adhesive tape
pencil
yellow paper
glue
black paint
paintbrush

FOR THE FACE
make-up sponge
water-based face paints
medium make-up brush

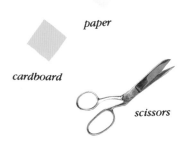
adhesive tape

paintbrush

glue   *ribbon*

paper

cardboard

scissors

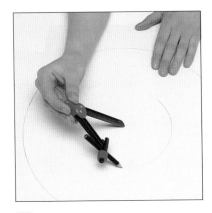

1 To make the costume, use a pair of compasses to draw and cut out a circle from a piece of cardboard. Draw and cut out a circle in the middle big enough for your face to show through.

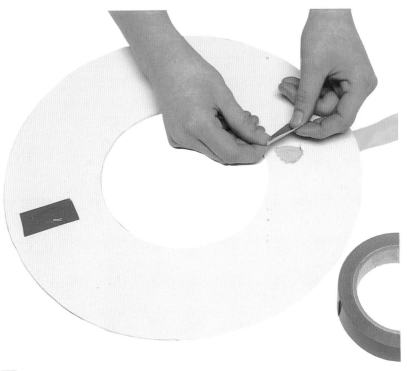

2 Make a slit either side of the circle and thread a piece of ribbon through. Secure the ribbon down with a knot and a piece of adhesive tape.

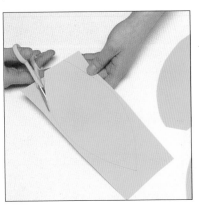

3 Draw a petal shape onto yellow paper, and use it as a template for the others. You will need about 42 petals for a full sunflower. Cut out the petals.

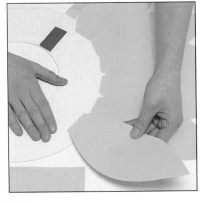

4 Starting at the edge of the cardboard circle, glue on the petals so that they overlap each other. When you have covered the outer edge start on the second row and finish off in the centre of the circle.

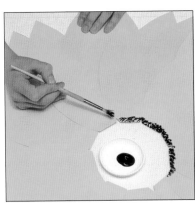

5 Paint black marks around the centre of the sunflower and leave the paint to dry. When you are ready to wear the flower, tie the ribbon around your head in a bow.

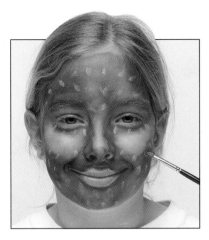

6 For the face, use a damp sponge to apply a brown base colour. Use a medium brush to paint yellow spots on the base colour. Paint the lips the same colour.

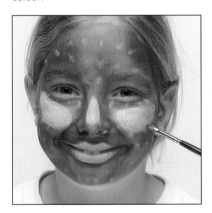

7 Paint yellow highlights under each eye and on the nose.

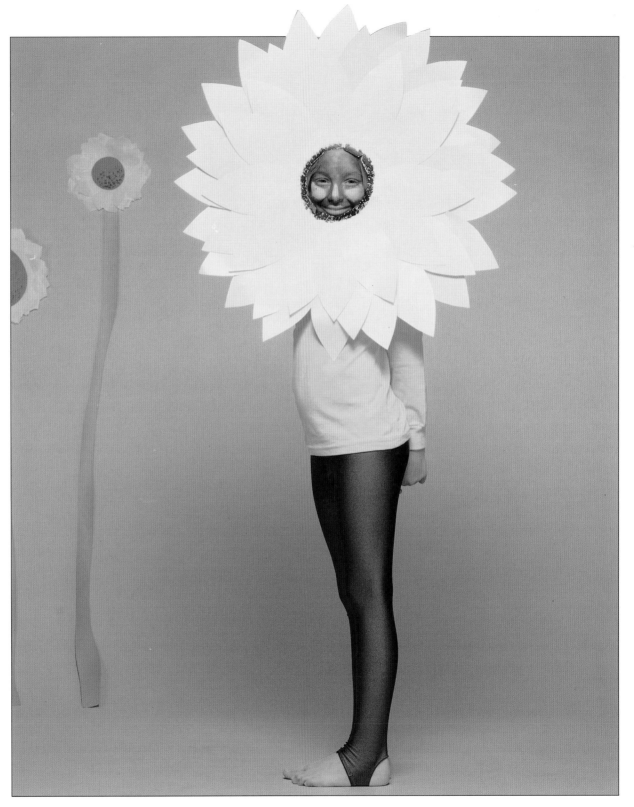

Pumpkin

You will certainly win the biggest pumpkin competition if you wear this outfit.

YOU WILL NEED
hairband
green paint
paintbrush
scissors
green fabric
needle and thread or sewing machine
stuffing (batting)
3 metres/3 yards orange fabric
fabric tape
milliner's wire
safety pin
elastic

hairband

thread

fabric

milliner's wire

elastic

scissors

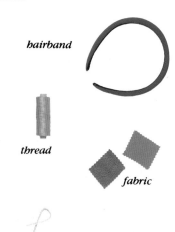

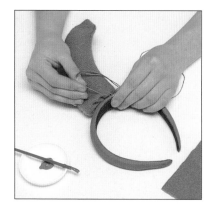

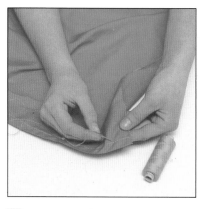

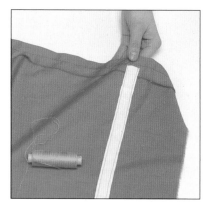

1 To make the pumpkin stalk, first paint the hairband green and leave it to dry. Cut out two pieces of fabric for the stalk and sew them together with the right sides facing. Leave a gap and turn right sides out. Fill the stalk with stuffing (batting) and sew up the end. Sew the stalk onto the centre of the hairband.

2 To make the pumpkin body, first fold over the two long sides of the orange fabric and sew a line of stitches on each long side to make a 1.5 cm/½ in tube for the elastic.

3 Sew lengths of fabric tape widthwise on the reverse side of the fabric. You will need to sew on approximately five lengths of tape, positioned equal distances apart.

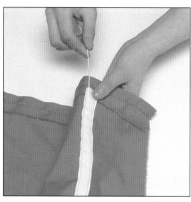

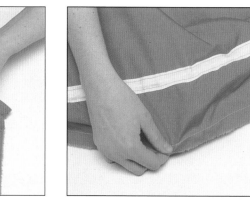

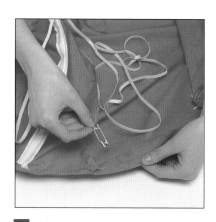

4 Thread a length of milliner's wire through each fabric tape tube. Bend the ends over and sew them onto the tape.

5 With the right sides facing fold the fabric in half widthwise, and turn so that the tubes for the elastic are at the top and bottom. Sew the shorter sides together.

6 Attach a safety pin to the elastic and thread through the top and bottom tubes. Pull the end of the elastic to gather the fabric and tie a double knot. Before you try on the pumpkin costume, bend the wires so that they are curved, to make a full, round shape.

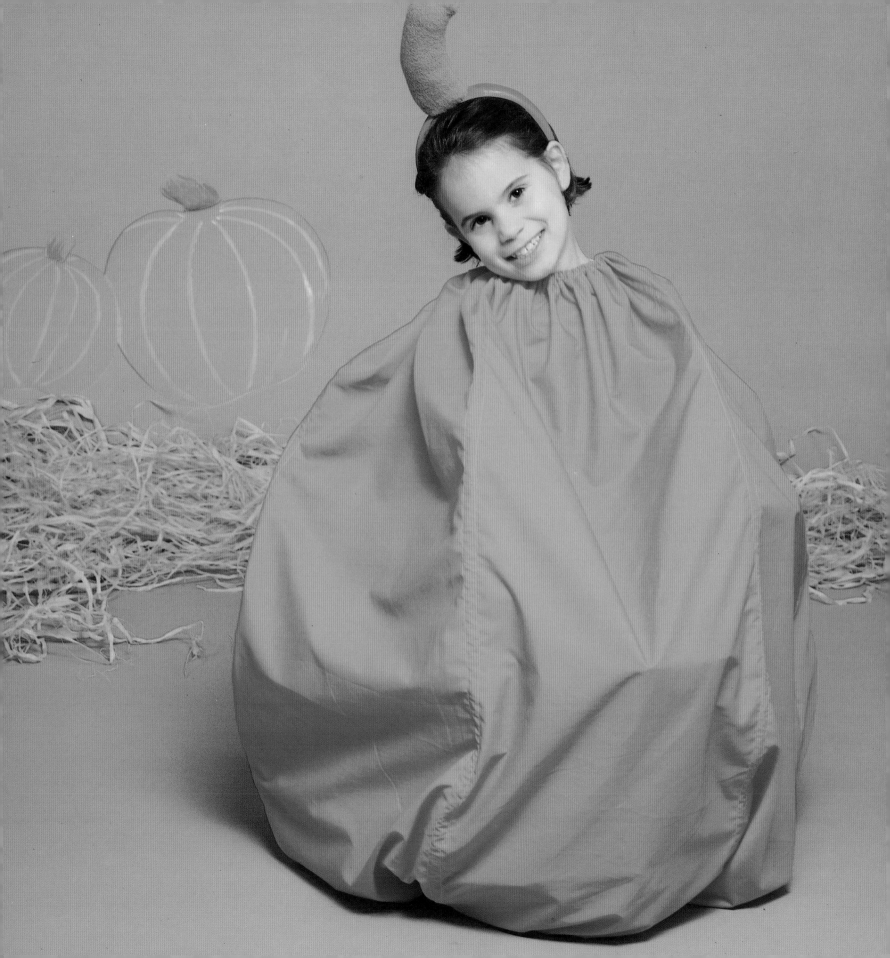

Carrot

For the complete outfit, dress up in an orange T-shirt and leggings and, if you have an old pair of shoes, paint them orange.

YOU WILL NEED
pencil
green cardboard
scissors
glue

FOR THE FACE
make-up sponge
water-based face paints

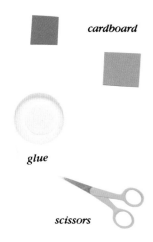
cardboard

glue

scissors

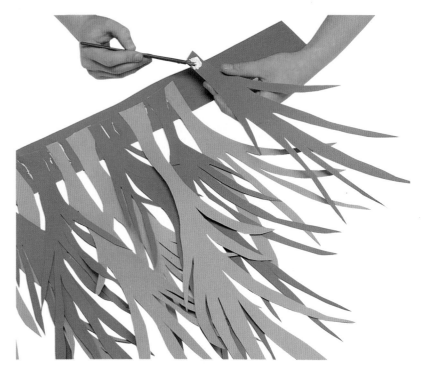

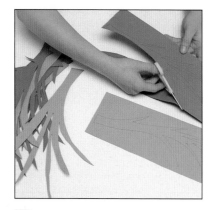

1 Draw lots of differently shaped leaves on green cardboard and cut them out.

2 Cut two strips of green cardboard 5 cm/2 in wide and long enough to fit around your head. Glue the leaves along one of the strips.

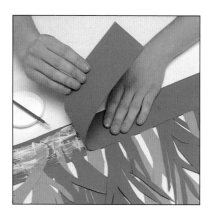

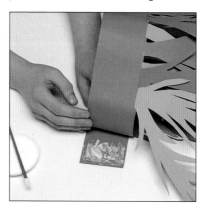

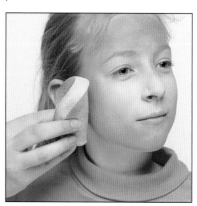

3 Glue the other strip on top of the first, sandwiching the base of the leaves between the two. Leave the glue to dry.

4 Curve the card to fit around your head and glue the two ends of the strip together. Leave the glue to dry before trying the headdress on.

5 For the face, use a make-up sponge to apply an orange base all over.

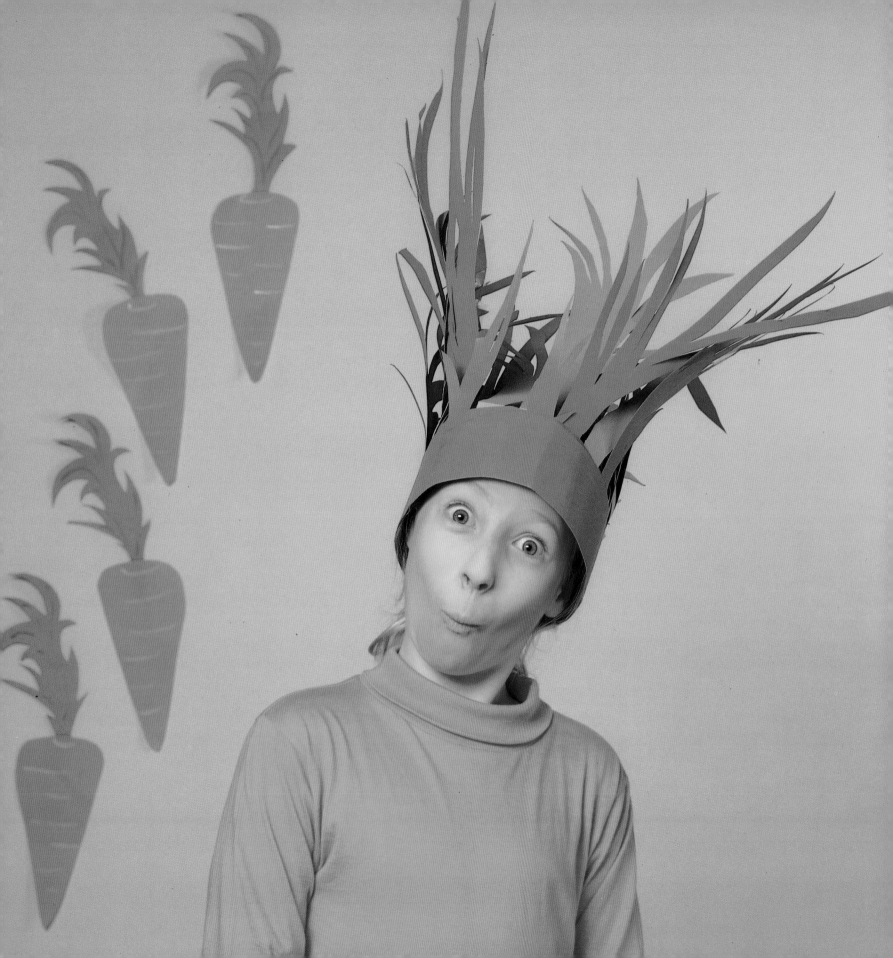

Genie

You can make your own baggy pantaloons by following the instructions provided in the introduction.

YOU WILL NEED
pair of shoes
glitter paint
paintbrush
glue
glittery braid
scraps of fabric
baggy trousers (pants) or pantaloons
scissors
fabric glue
fabric for the cummerbund
tape measure
needle and thread or sewing machine
fabric for the turban
feathers

FOR THE FACE
make-up sponge
water-based face paints
medium make-up brush

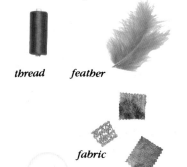

thread   *feather*

fabric

fabric glue

glittery braid

paintbrush

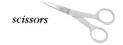

scissors

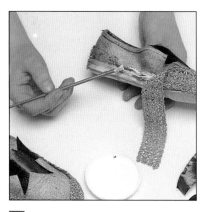

1 To make the costume, paint a pair of shoes a sparkling colour and leave to dry. Stick a piece of glittery braid around the side of each shoe.

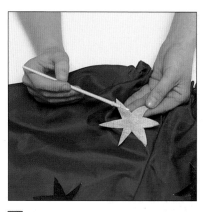

2 Making use of scraps of fabric, cut out lots of stars and glue them onto a pair of baggy trousers (pants) or pantaloons using fabric glue.

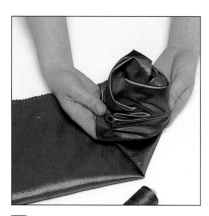

3 Measure your waist for the cummerbund, allowing an extra 25 cm/10 in so you can tie the fabric at the back. Sew two pieces of fabric together to the required length with the right sides facing, leaving an opening at one end, and turn it right side out. Sew up the end.

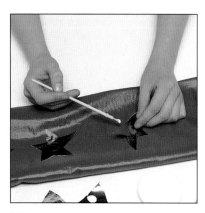

4 Cut out some more stars from scraps of fabric and glue them onto the cummerbund with fabric glue.

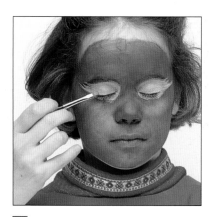

5 For the face, use a damp sponge to apply the base colour, avoiding the area around the eyes. Paint the area around the eyes a bright colour.

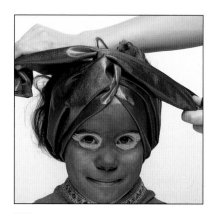

6 Tie the turban around the head, tying a knot on the top of the head. Tuck the loose fabric underneath the turban. Place a few colourful feathers on the top of the turban to decorate.

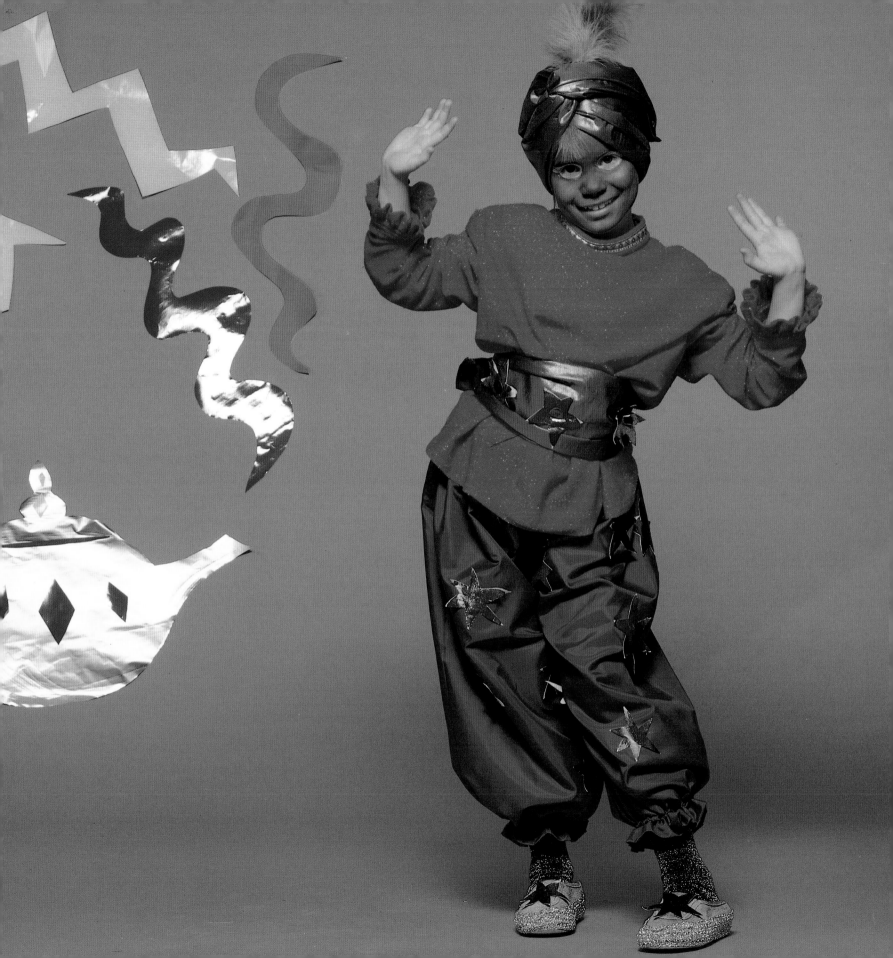

Dragon

To make a pair of ears follow the instructions provided
for the devil horns.

YOU WILL NEED
red fabric
scissors
needle and thread
pair of children's red tights
newspaper or stuffing (batting)
elastic

FOR THE FACE
make-up sponge
water-based face paints
stipple sponge
medium make-up brush

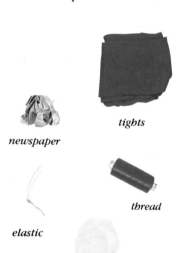

newspaper

tights

elastic

thread

stuffing (batting)

scissors

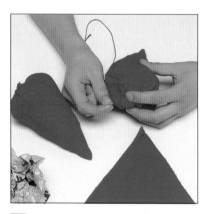

1 To make the tail, cut two triangles of fabric for each spike. Sew them together, leaving one side open. Fill each spike with crumpled-up newspaper or stuffing (batting). Sew a running stitch around the opening and pull the threads to gather up the end. Tie a knot to secure.

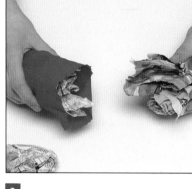

2 Cut one leg off the tights and fill it with crumpled-up newspaper. Sew up the end and pull the thread tight.

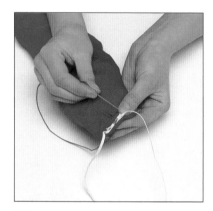

3 Sew a loop of elastic to the end of the tail, long enough to fit comfortably around your waist.

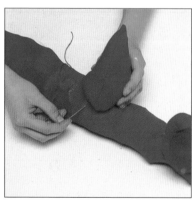

4 Sew the spikes onto the tail.

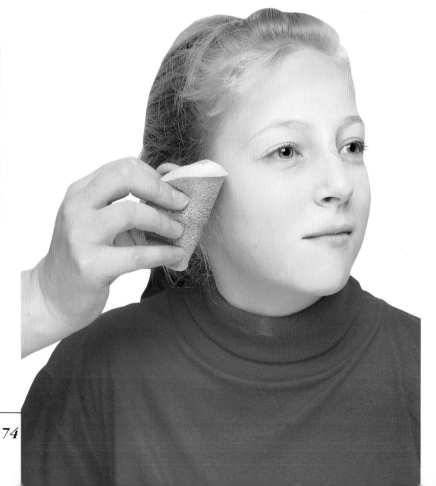

5 For the face, use a damp make-up sponge to apply a base colour.

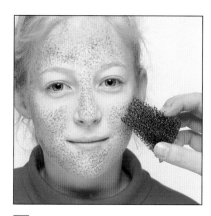

6 Using a stipple sponge, stipple a dark colour on the base, avoiding the area around the eyes and the mouth.

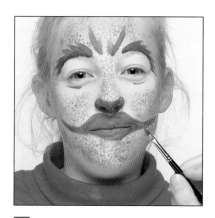

7 Using a medium brush, paint a large mouth, eyebrows, the tip of the nose and marks on the forehead.

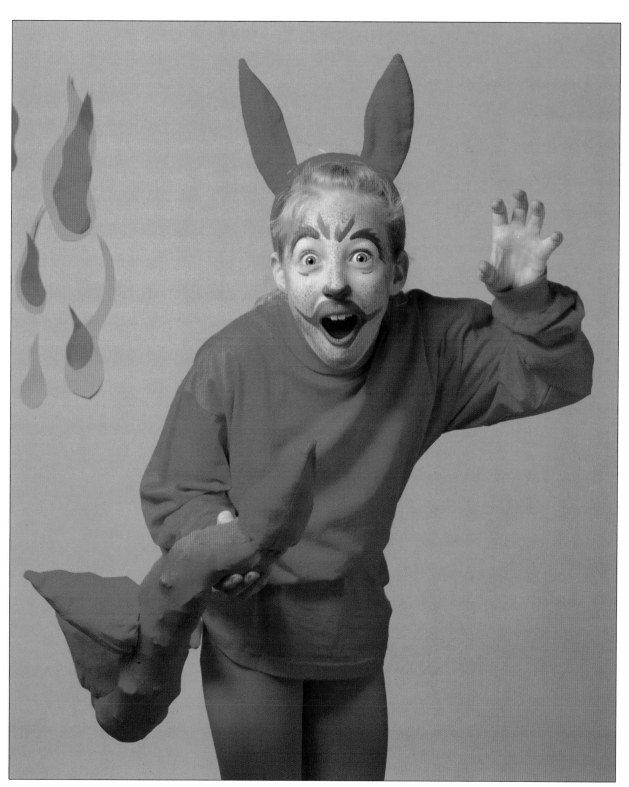

Gypsy

Wear your brightest clothes to go with the accessories and make up your own gypsy dance.

YOU WILL NEED
cardboard
scissors
newspaper
PVA (white) glue
bowl
water
paints
paintbrush
glitter
sequins
fabric for the head scarf and shawl
needle and thread or sewing machine
braid
pom-poms

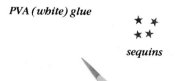

braid

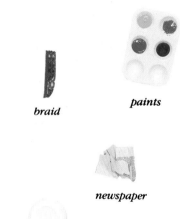

paints

newspaper

PVA (white) glue

sequins

scissors

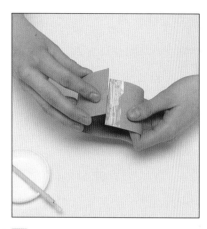

1 Cut a strip of cardboard to fit comfortably around your wrist and approximately 5 cm/2 in wide. Bend the cardboard to make a bracelet and glue it in place.

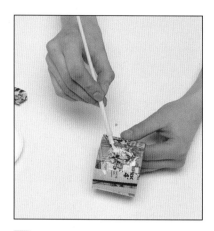

2 Scrunch up small balls of newspaper and glue them onto the bracelet. Cover the bangle in three layers of papier mâché as described in the introduction, and leave it to dry thoroughly in a warm place.

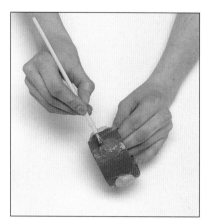

3 Paint the bangle using lots of colours and leave the paint to dry.

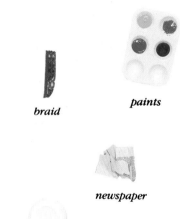

4 Paint dabs of glue on the bangle and sprinkle on the glitter. Glue a few sequins on for extra sparkle and decoration. Leave the glue to dry before trying on the bracelet.

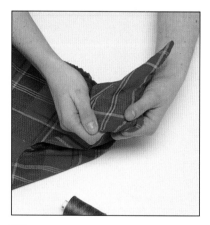

5 For the head scarf, sew two triangular pieces of fabric together with the right sides facing. Leave a gap and turn right side out. Sew up the gap.

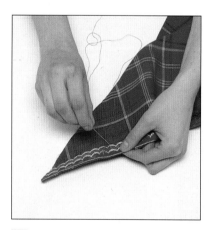

6 Sew a strip of braid along the longest side of the scarf. Make a larger, but similar, scarf to go around the neck and sew pom-poms along the sides.

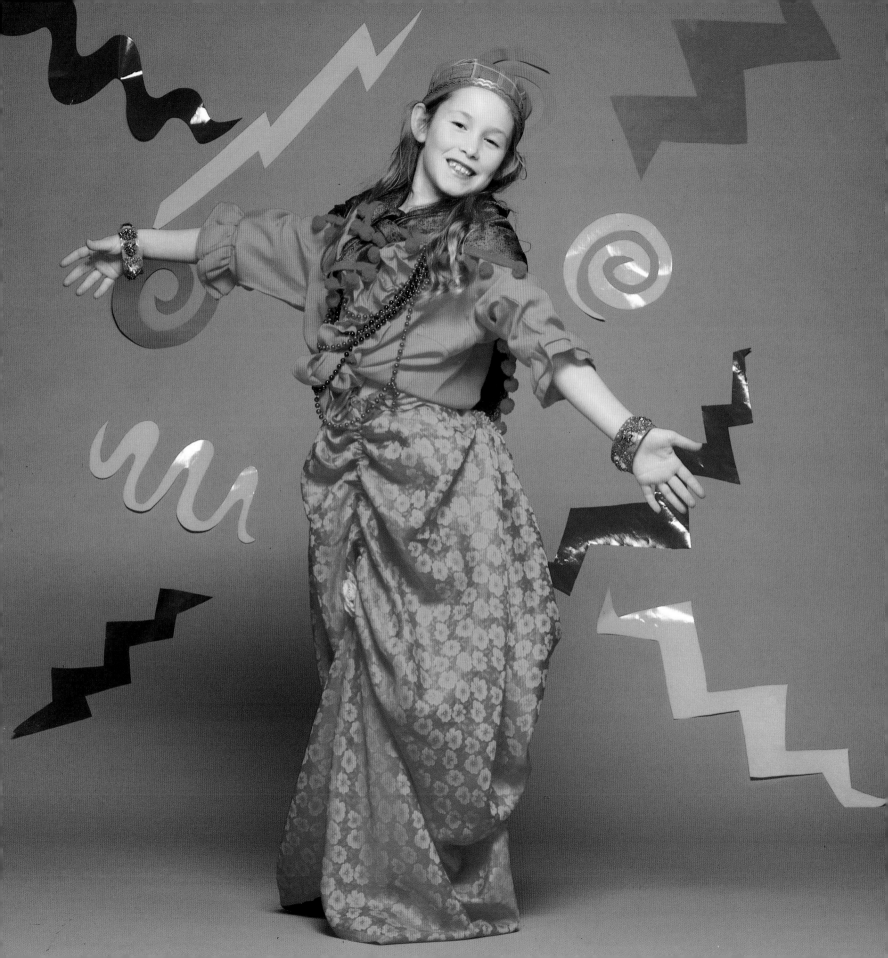

Cowboy

Find a hat and a toy gun to complete this costume. Round up your friends and have fun.

YOU WILL NEED
tape measure
felt for the waistcoat (vest)
scissors
needle and thread or sewing machine
templates for pocket
pins
fabric glue
template for sheriff badge
pencil
cardboard
tin foil or silver paint
paintbrush
safety pin
strong adhesive tape

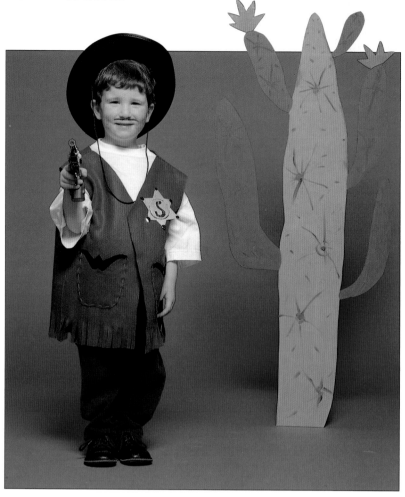

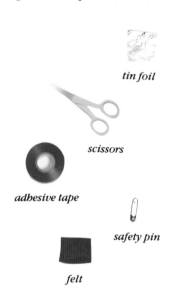

tin foil

scissors

adhesive tape

safety pin

felt

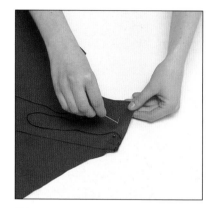

1 For the waistcoat (vest), measure from the nape of your neck to the length required, and cut two squares of felt to this size. Cut one piece in half lengthways for the two front pieces. With the right sides facing, sew the two front pieces to the back along the shoulders. Sew the sides together leaving gaps for the arms.

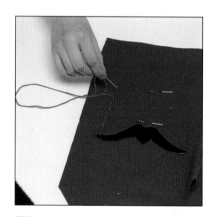

2 Turn the waistcoat right side out. Use the template to cut out two pockets from felt. Pin them in position on the front. Use the template to cut out two pieces of fabric in a contrasting colour to decorate the top of each pocket and glue them on with fabric glue. Sew the pockets onto the waistcoat using brightly coloured thread.

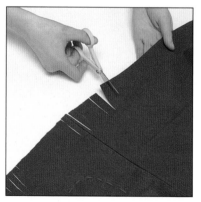

3 Using a pair of scissors, snip along the bottom of the waistcoat to make a fringe.

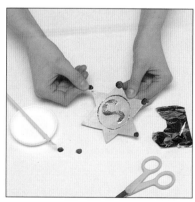

4 To make the badge, use the template to draw around and cut out a piece of cardboard and cover it in tin foil or paint it silver. Decorate the badge with a silver "S" in the centre and silver spots on the tip of each point. Fasten a safety pin onto the reverse of the badge with a piece of tape.

Native American

You can buy the feathers for this costume from most good fabric shops. You can make the skirt from felt with an elastic waistband.

YOU WILL NEED
tape measure
wide ribbon
scissors
feathers
felt
fabric glue
needle and embroidery threads
wool
narrow ribbon

FOR THE FACE
water-based face paints
medium make-up brush

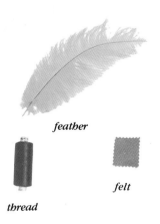
feather

thread

felt

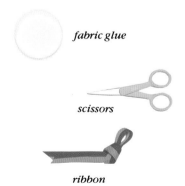
fabric glue

scissors

ribbon

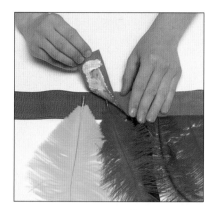

1 Measure around your head with a tape measure, allowing a 5 cm/2 in overlap and cut the wide ribbon to this length. Arrange the feathers in the centre of the ribbon on the reverse side. Cut a strip of felt the same width as the ribbon and glue it onto the feathers. This will help to secure them in place.

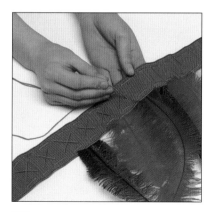

2 Sew a few lines of decorative stitching along the ribbon, using colourful embroidery threads. With the right sides facing, sew the two ends of the ribbon together.

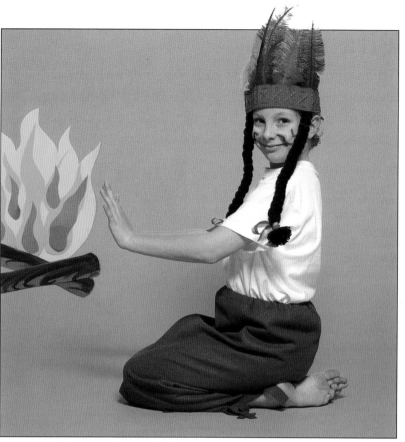

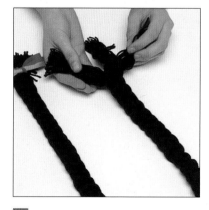

3 To make each plait (braid), you will need approximately 45 equal strands of wool. Tie a piece of wool around one end of each bundle. Ask a friend to help you with the plaiting by holding one end of the bundle tight while you plait. Tie a piece of ribbon in a bow at the end of each plait.

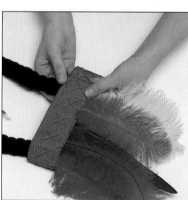

4 Sew or glue the plaits onto the inside of the headdress, so that they lie either side of your face. For the face, use bright colours to paint three zig-zag lines on each cheek.

Pirate

This young pirate is dressed for an exciting and adventurous voyage across the ocean. Glue a skull and crossbones onto a plain T-shirt and tie a scarf around your neck to complete the costume.

YOU WILL NEED
black felt
scissors
template for skull and crossbones
pencil
white felt
fabric glue
needle and thread
elastic
pins

FOR THE FACE
fine make-up brush
water-based face paints

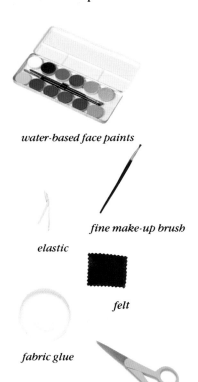

water-based face paints

fine make-up brush

elastic

felt

fabric glue

scissors

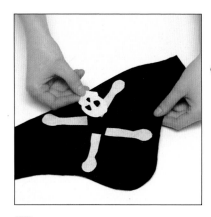

1 For the hat, cut two equal pieces of fabric, following the shape in the photograph. Using the template for the skull and crossbones draw around and cut out the shapes from white felt. Glue them onto the front of the hat with fabric glue.

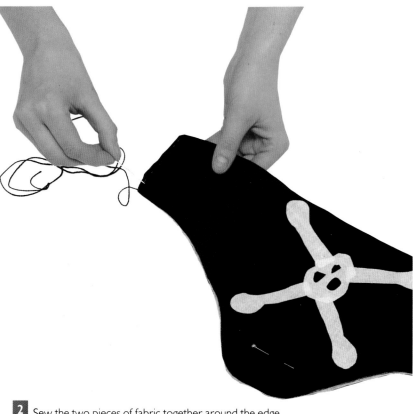

2 Sew the two pieces of fabric together around the edge.

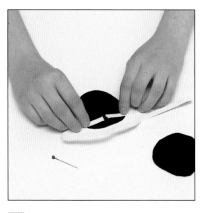

3 To make the eye patch, cut out two pieces of black felt the same size. Cut a piece of elastic long enough to go around your head. Trap the elastic in between the two patches and pin in place.

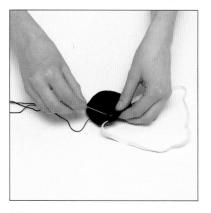

4 Sew around the edge of the patch to secure the elastic.

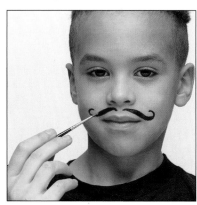

5 For the face, use a fine make-up brush to paint on a moustache.

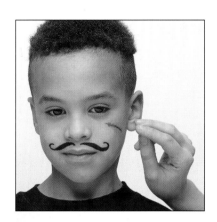

6 Use your fingertips to rub on red and purple to make a bruised scar.

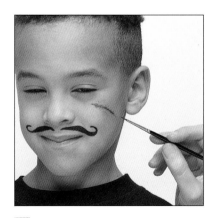

7 Paint a line down the centre of the scar with a fine brush.

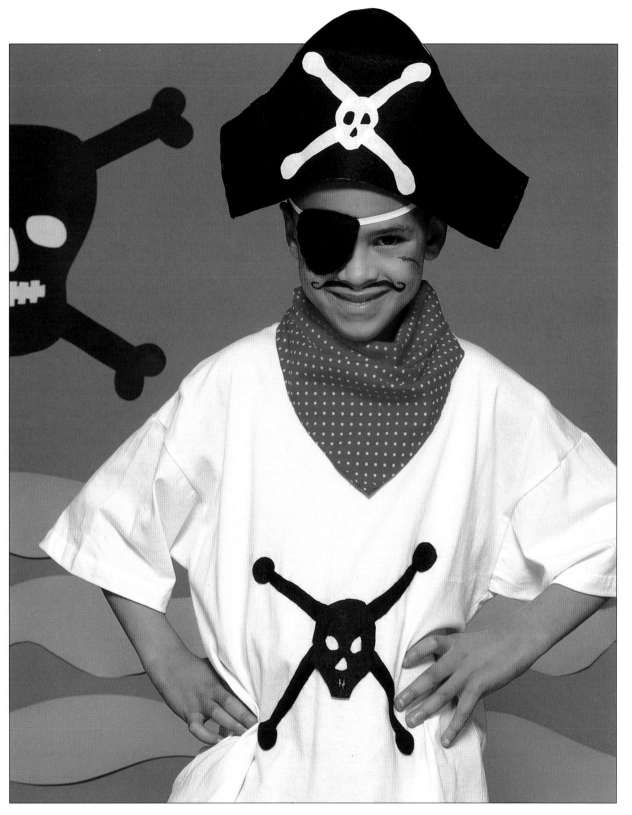

Prince

To make a sword, follow the instructions given for the knight's costume. The cloak was made from a piece of fabric found at a flea market and was decorated with a piece of tinsel to match the crown.

YOU WILL NEED
tape measure
pencil
scissors
cardboard
silver paint
paintbrush
coloured foil paper
glue
glitter
tinsel
fabric for cloak
safety pins

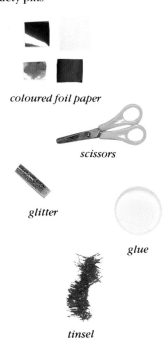

coloured foil paper

scissors

glitter

glue

tinsel

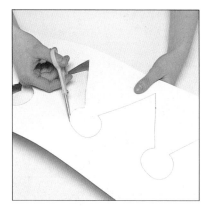

1 Measure around your head with a tape measure so that you know approximately how big to make the crown. Draw and cut out the crown from a piece of cardboard.

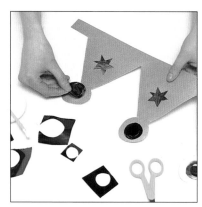

2 Paint the cardboard silver and leave the paint to dry thoroughly. Cut shapes out of coloured foil paper and glue them onto the crown. Paint dots of glue onto the shapes and sprinkle on some glitter.

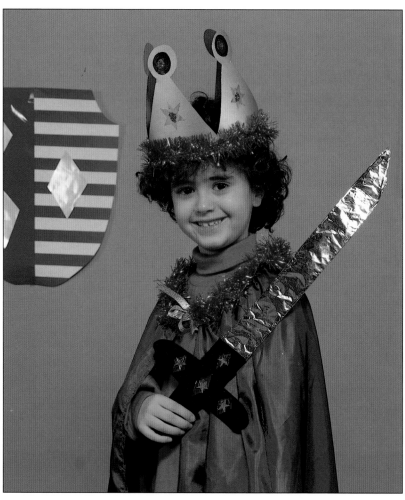

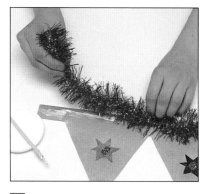

3 Glue a piece of tinsel around the rim of the crown and leave the glue to dry.

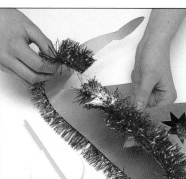

4 Glue the two ends of the crown together to fit on your head and leave the glue to dry before you try the crown on. Pin the fabric to your shoulders to make a cloak.

Princess

If you have always dreamed of being a beautiful young princess, and imagined living in a castle, dress up in this costume and maybe your dream will come true.

YOU WILL NEED
tape measure
fabric for hat
fabric interfacing (optional)
pencil
scissors
needle and thread
chiffon fabric
wool
narrow ribbon
braid

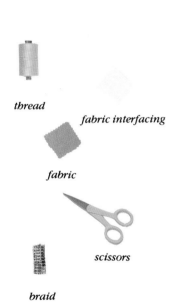

thread

fabric interfacing

fabric

scissors

braid

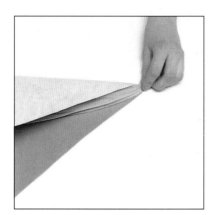

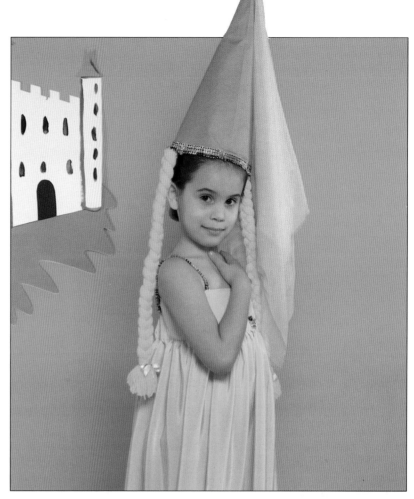

1 Measure the width of your head with a tape measure, so that you know how wide to make the rim of the hat. If the fabric you are using needs to be stiffened, iron a piece of interfacing onto the reverse side. Draw and cut out a triangle with a curved base, making sure the rim measures the width of your head, with an allowance for sewing together. Sew a hem around the rim of the triangle and, with the right sides facing, fold the triangle in half, trapping a piece of chiffon fabric at the point of the cone.

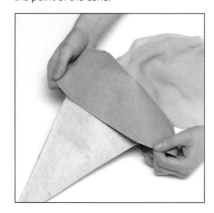

2 Sew the cone together and turn it right side out.

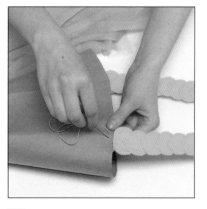

3 Following the instructions for the Native American, make a pair of woollen plaits (braids) and tie a piece of ribbon in a bow around the end of each one. Sew the plaits onto the inside of the hat, so that they lie either side of the face.

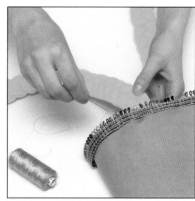

4 Sew a piece of braid around the rim of the hat, and arrange the chiffon fabric so that it trails down the side like a veil.

Hippy

Be loving and laid-back in this colourful flower-power costume. Search local flea markets and second-hand shops for bright clothes to wear with the accessories. Go completely wild and paint a flower on your cheek.

YOU WILL NEED
template for flower pendant
pencil
scissors
cardboard
newspaper
PVA (white) glue
bowl
water
paints
paintbrush
hole puncher
ribbon
fabric or old scarf
scraps of coloured felt
needle and thread
buttons
tissue and crepe paper
garden canes

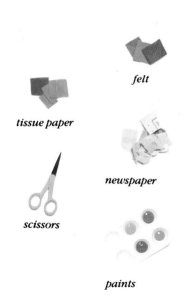

felt

tissue paper

newspaper

scissors

paints

 buttons

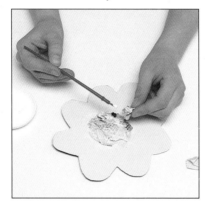

1 Use the template to draw around and cut a piece of cardboard in the shape of a flower. Scrunch up small balls of newspaper and glue them in the centre of the flower.

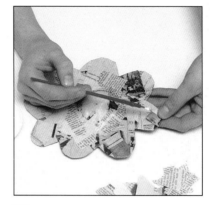

2 Cover the flower in three layers of papier mâché as described in the introduction and leave to dry thoroughly in a warm place.

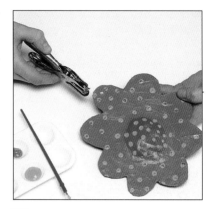

3 Paint the flower in lots of bright colours and leave to dry. Using a hole puncher, punch a hole in one of the petals and thread a piece of ribbon through.

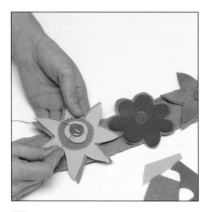

4 For the headband you will need a band of bright fabric or an old scarf. Cut out different shaped flowers from coloured felt. Sew the flowers onto the headband and sew a button onto the centre of each flower.

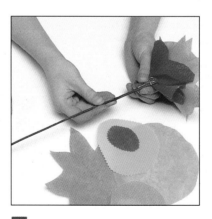

5 To make a colourful bouquet of flowers, first cut out lots of shapes in tissue and crepe paper. Starting with the largest petal at the bottom, layer the petals on top of each other, piercing a hole through them with the garden cane.

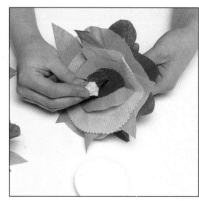

6 Roll a piece of tissue paper with glue and place it in the centre of the flower on the stick. Fan out the petals to finish off.

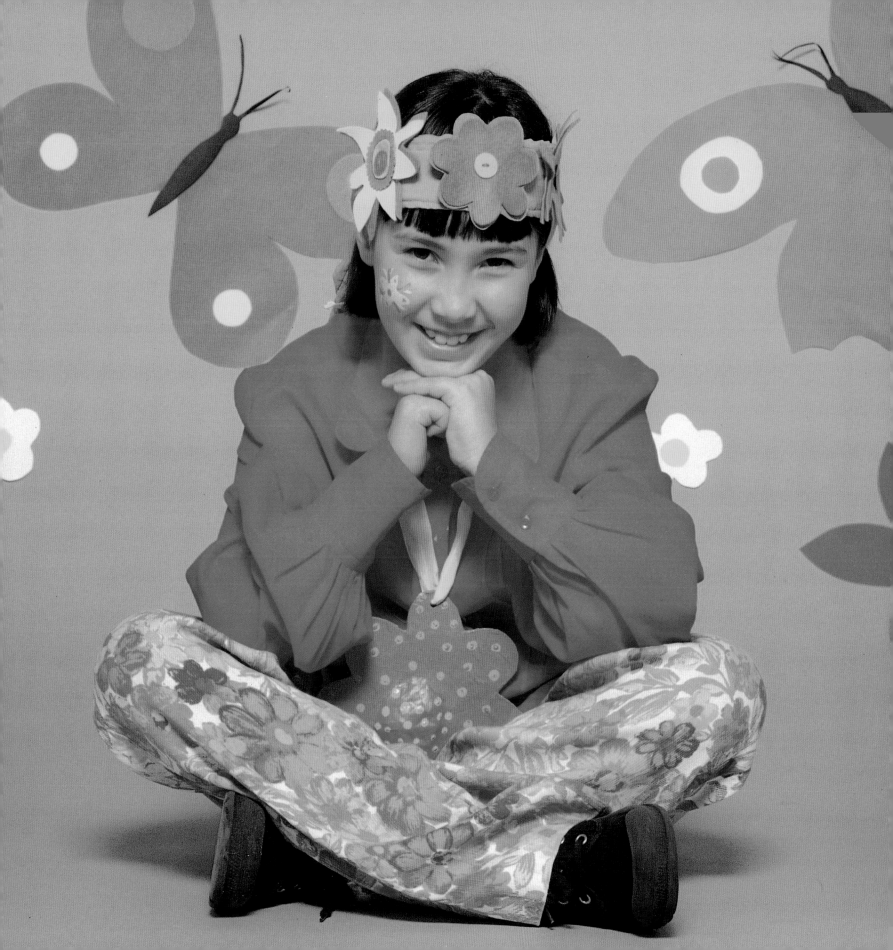

Knight

Have a pretend battle with your friends in this shiny suit of armour.

YOU WILL NEED
cardboard
scissors
tin foil
black felt
glue
coloured foil paper
template for helmet
pencil
silver paint
paintbrush
template for body shield
hole puncher
ribbon

paint

glue

scissors

coloured foil paper

tin foil

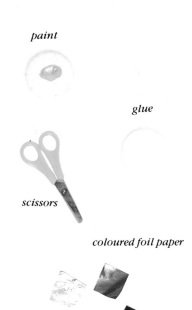

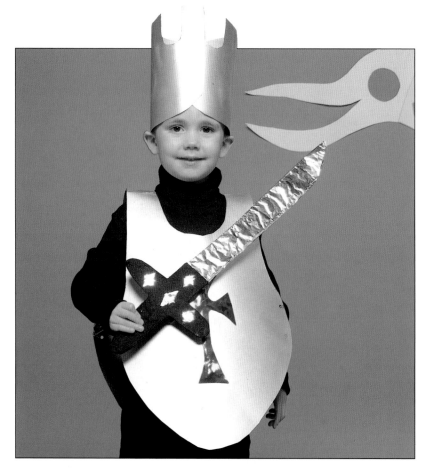

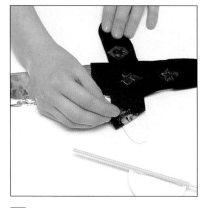

1 Cut a piece of cardboard in the shape of a sword. Cover the blade in silver foil. Cut two pieces of felt to fit the handle of the sword and glue them on. Decorate the handle with diamond shapes cut out of foil paper.

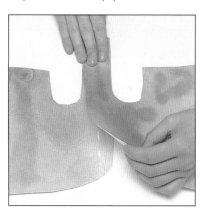

2 To make the helmet, use the template to draw and cut two equal pieces of cardboard. Paint these silver and leave to dry. Glue the two pieces together as shown in the picture.

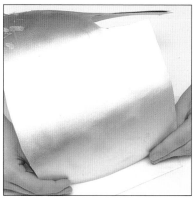

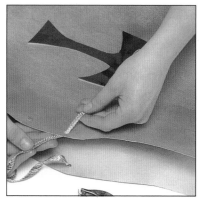

3 When the glue has dried, fold the helmet so that it curves and glue the sides together. Hold the helmet together while the glue dries. To make the body shield you will need to draw round the shape, then flip it to complete the other half. Do this for the front and back pieces and cut them out.

4 Paint the two pieces silver. When the paint has dried, glue the two pieces together at the shoulder seam. Cut a foil paper cross and glue it onto the front of the shield. Punch a hole on either side of the body shield and thread a piece of ribbon through. Tie a knot to secure.

Wizard

Wave the magic wand and conjure up some secret spells. Look in flea markets for a piece of material to make the cape.

YOU WILL NEED
tape measure
fabric for hat
fabric interfacing (optional)
scissors
needle and thread
silver fabric
fabric glue
templates for wizard's pendant
pencil
cardboard
tin foil
silver ribbon
double-sided adhesive tape
garden cane
paint
paintbrush
tinsel

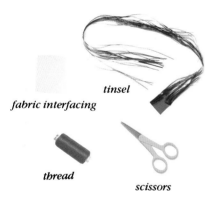

tinsel

fabric interfacing

thread

scissors

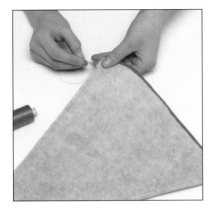

1 Measure the width of your head with a tape measure so that you know how wide to make the rim of the hat. If the fabric you are using needs to be stiffened, iron a piece of interfacing onto the reverse side. Ask an adult to help you. Draw and cut out a triangle with a curved base, making sure the rim measures the width of your head with a small allowance for sewing together. Hem the bottom and, with right sides facing, fold the triangle in half to make a tall cone. Sew along the side. Turn the hat the right side out and decorate with silver fabric stars, stuck on with fabric glue.

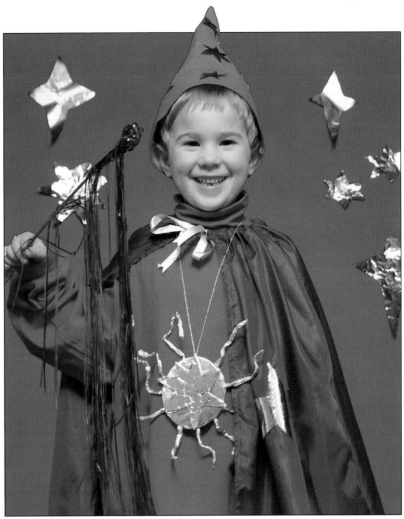

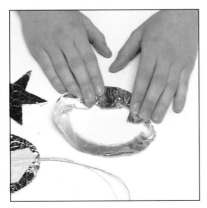

2 To make the pendant, use the template to cut out a cardboard star. Cut two circles of cardboard of the same size to make the backing. Cover both circles and the star with tin foil. Attach the ribbon to the back of the card circles with a piece of adhesive tape.

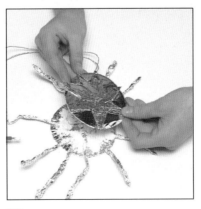

3 Roll up strips of foil and place them on the reverse of one of the foil circles. Glue the other circle on top to trap the foil strips and secure them in place.

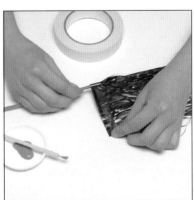

4 To make the wand, first paint a garden cane and leave it to dry. Stick a piece of shiny tinsel around one end of the stick with adhesive tape.

Super Hero

Be a hero for a day and make your very own costume.

YOU WILL NEED
cardboard
scissors
tin foil
coloured foil paper
glue
silver cardboard
ribbon
adhesive tape
leotard or catsuit
 2 metres/2 yards fabric
needle and thread

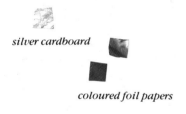
silver cardboard

coloured foil papers

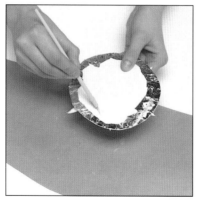
scissors

glue

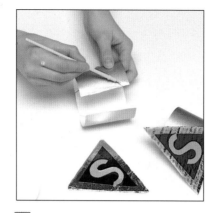

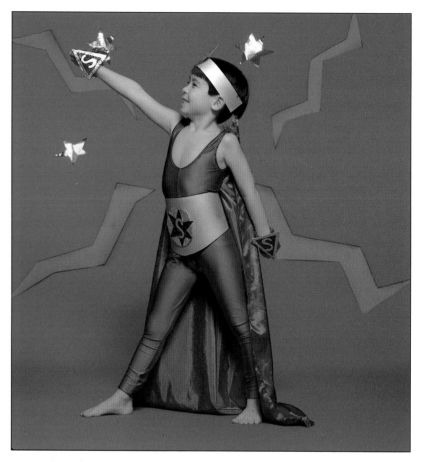

1 To make a wristband, first cut out a cardboard triangle and cover it in tin foil. Cut a smaller triangle in coloured foil paper and glue it onto the silver triangle. Cut out the letter "S" in silver cardboard and glue it onto the coloured triangle. Cut a strip of silver cardboard 5 cm/2 in wide and long enough to fit around your wrist. Glue the two ends together to make a band and glue on the triangle. Make another wristband the same way.

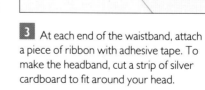

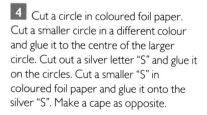

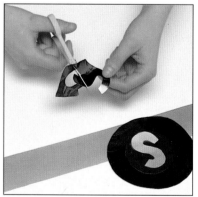

2 To make the waistband, cut a piece of cardboard to fit around your waist. Cut a circle from cardboard and cover it in tin foil. Cut a star from coloured foil paper and glue it onto the silver circle. Cut out the letter "S" in cardboard and glue it onto the star. Glue the circle onto the waistband.

3 At each end of the waistband, attach a piece of ribbon with adhesive tape. To make the headband, cut a strip of silver cardboard to fit around your head.

4 Cut a circle in coloured foil paper. Cut a smaller circle in a different colour and glue it to the centre of the larger circle. Cut out a silver letter "S" and glue it on the circles. Cut a smaller "S" in coloured foil paper and glue it onto the silver "S". Make a cape as opposite.

Super Heroine

Impress your friends and family with your heroic powers and dress up in this futuristic costume.

YOU WILL NEED
cardboard
scissors
tin foil
coloured foil paper
glue
silver cardboard
ribbon
adhesive tape
coloured cardboard (optional)
leotard or catsuit
2 metres/2 yards fabric
needle and thread

scissors

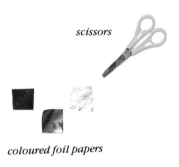

coloured foil papers

glue

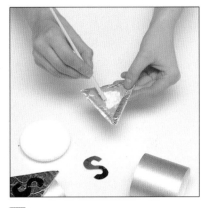

1 Make the wristband, waistband and headband as for the Super Hero's outfit.

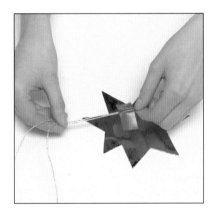

2 To make the pendant, cut out a star in silver or coloured cardboard and glue the letter "S" onto it. On the back of the star, attach a piece of ribbon in a loop with strong adhesive tape.

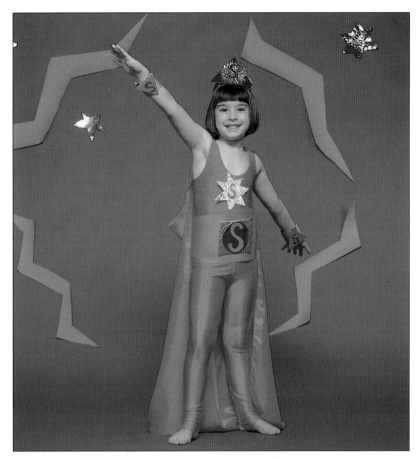

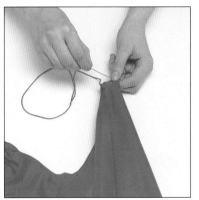

3 To make the cloak you will need a leotard or catsuit. Sew one end of the fabric onto the leotard shoulder straps.

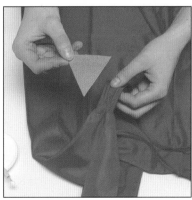

4 Where the fabric joins the straps, glue on silver cardboard triangles.

TEMPLATES

Some of the projects in this book need templates. You can either
trace them directly from the book, or enlarge them to the size
required. To double the size of a template, make a grid twice as large
as the one below. For instance, if one square equals 2.5 cm/1 in, then
draw a grid with 5 cm/2 in squares. Then copy the diagram square by
square. If you wish to make the template larger still, simply enlarge
the grid accordingly.

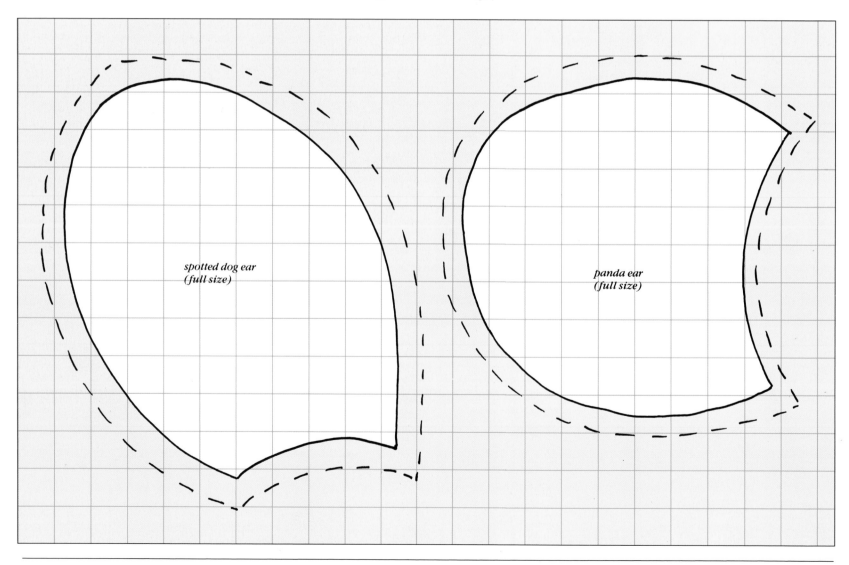

spotted dog ear
(full size)

panda ear
(full size)

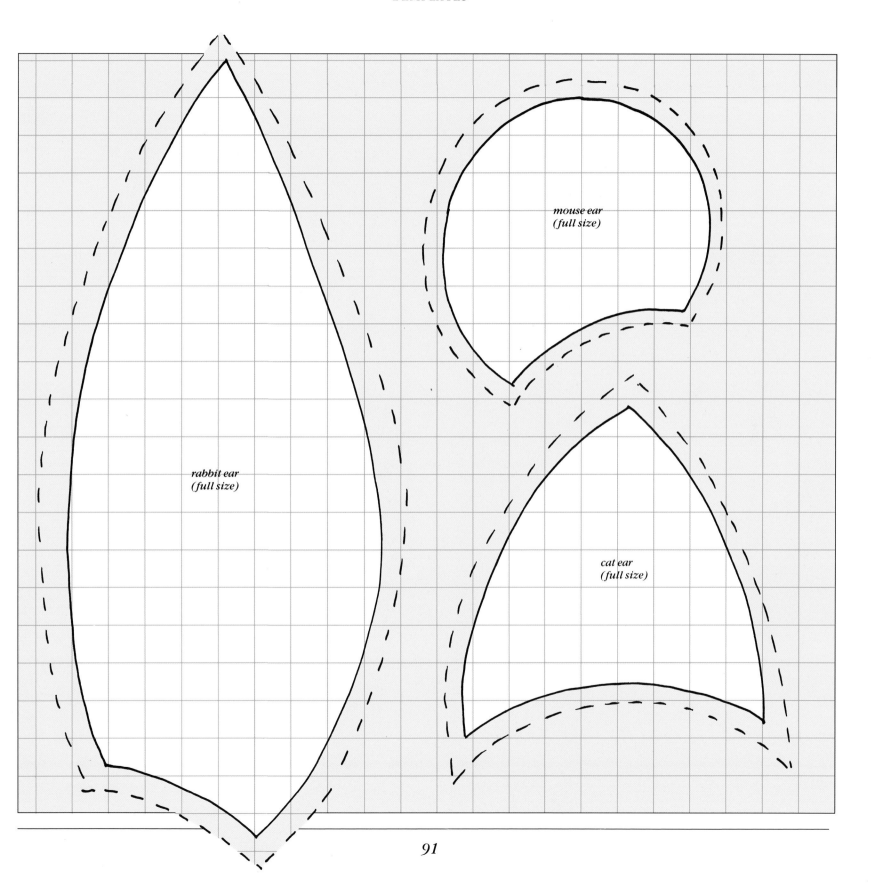

mouse ear
(full size)

rabbit ear
(full size)

cat ear
(full size)

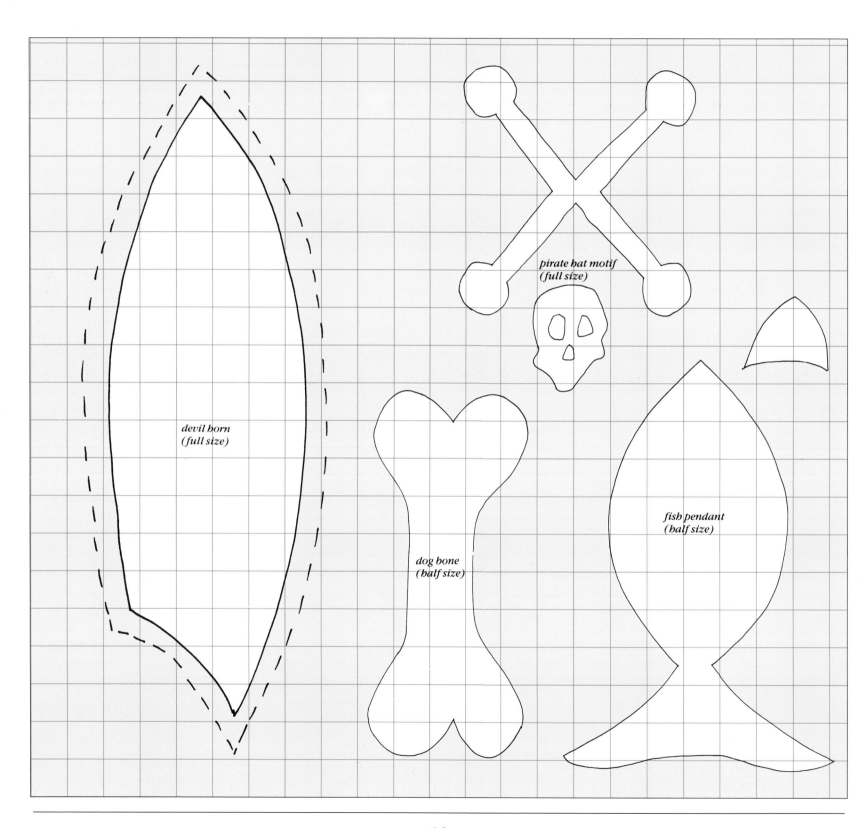

pirate hat motif
(full size)

devil horn
(full size)

dog bone
(half size)

fish pendant
(half size)

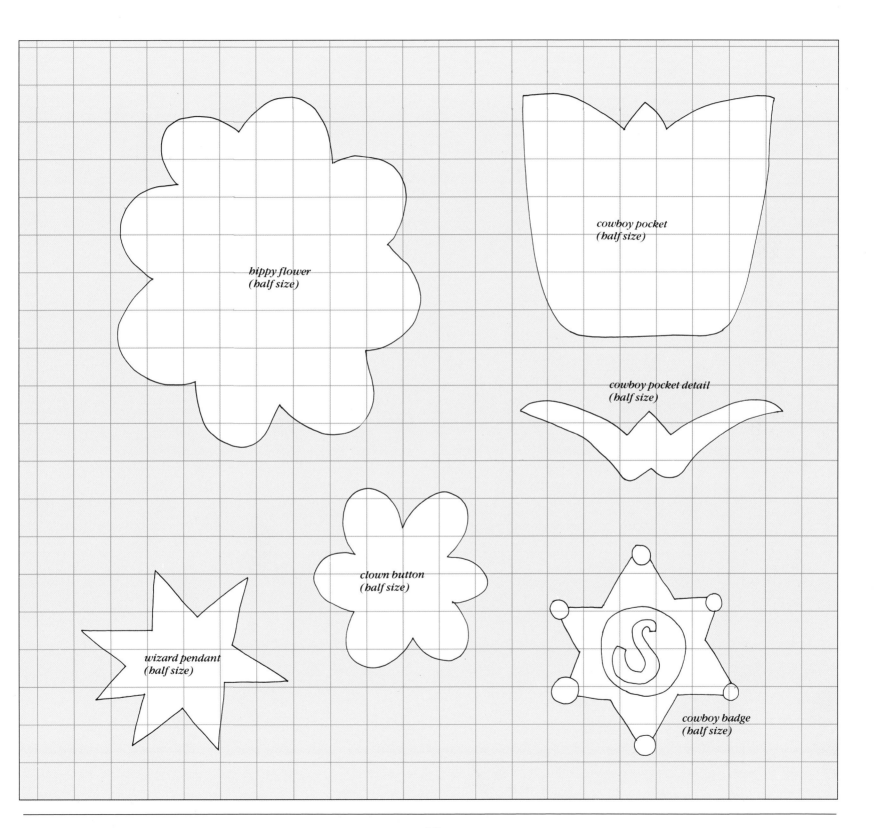

hippy flower
(half size)

cowboy pocket
(half size)

cowboy pocket detail
(half size)

clown button
(half size)

wizard pendant
(half size)

cowboy badge
(half size)

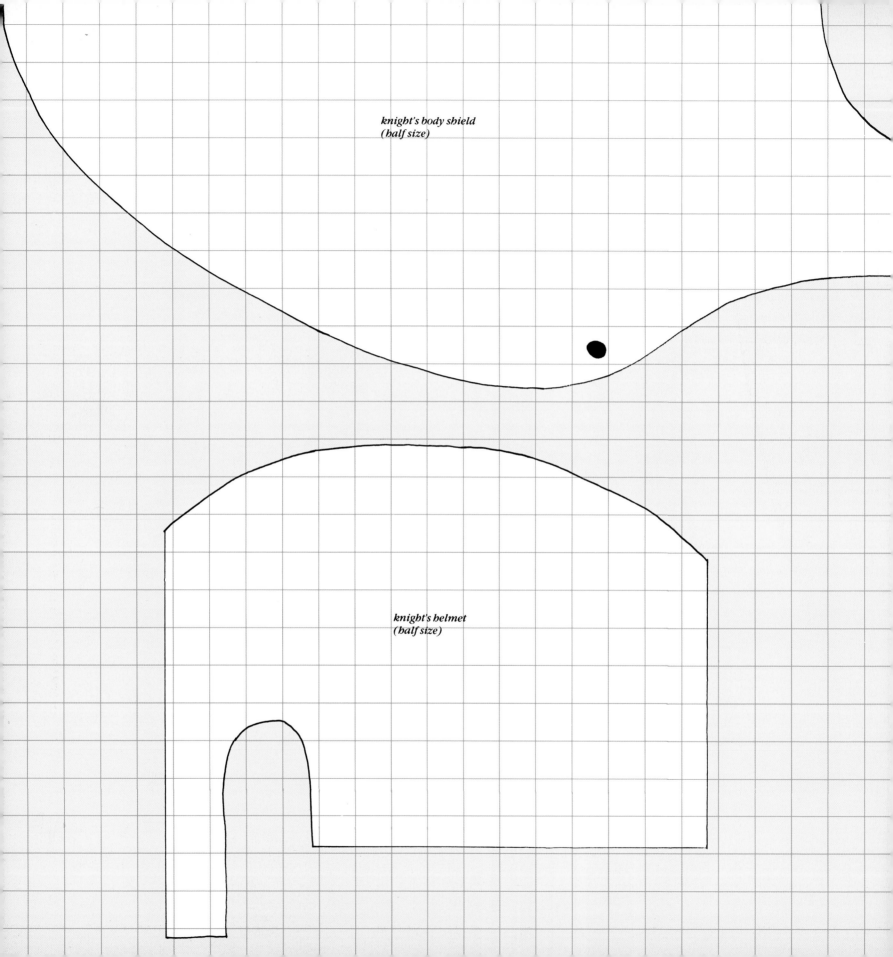

knight's body shield
(half size)

knight's helmet
(half size)

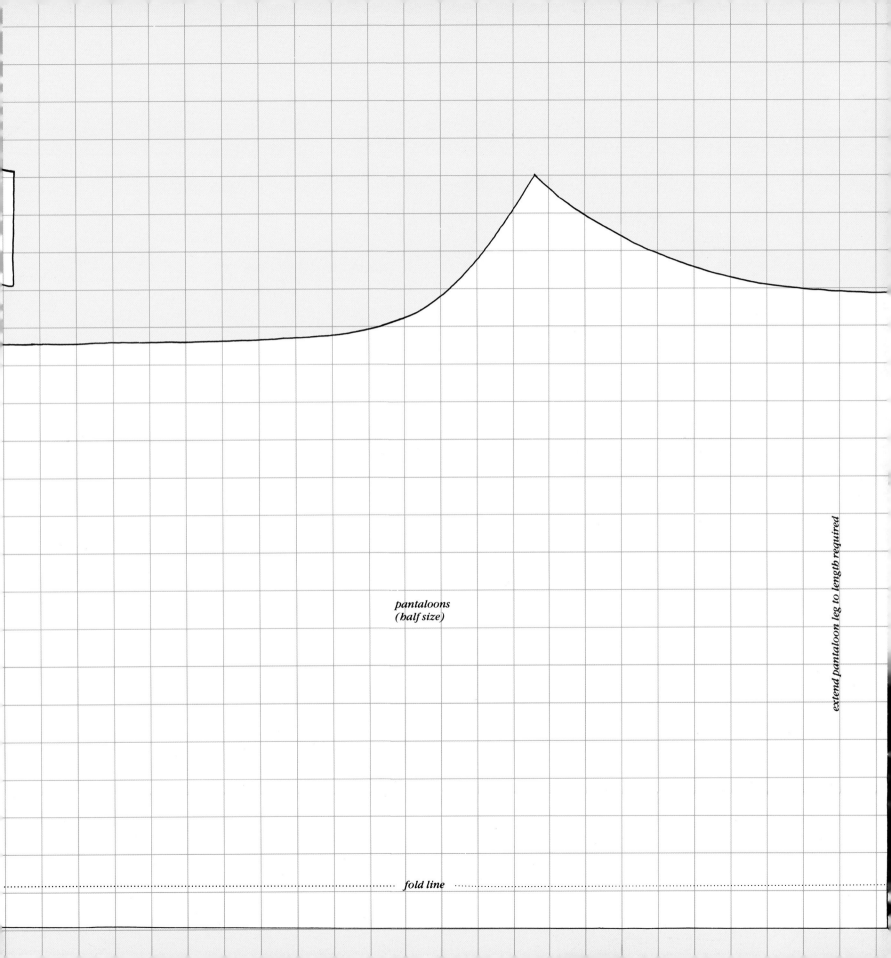

pantaloons
(half size)

extend pantaloon leg to length required

fold line

INDEX

ACKNOWLEDGEMENTS

The author and publishers would like to thank the following models and their parents for their contribution.

Alex, Alice, Anthony, Clare, Faye, Helen, Jade, Jessica, Joe, Joshua, Kelly, Kirsty, Lucy, Otis, Patrick, Rosie, Sophy, Tanya, Timothy, Zoë and Zosia.

Special thanks to Screenface, 24 Powis Terrace, London W11 1JH for providing the pots of make-up in the Fardel range on page 11.

The author and publishers would also like to thank Caroline Thompson for her help in the studio.